The Circulation of Blood

A History

The Circulation of Blood

A History

Helen Rapson

Frederick Muller Limited
London

First published in Great Britain 1982 by
Frederick Muller Limited, London, SW19 7JU.

Copyright © 1982 by Helen Rapson

British Library Cataloguing in Publication Data

Rapson, Helen
   The circulation of blood—a history.
   1. Blood   2. Hematology—History
   I. Title
   612'.11'0722   QP91

   ISBN 0–584–11013–8

Phototypeset by Input Typesetting Ltd, London SW19 8DR
Printed in Great Britain by Redwood Burn Ltd, Trowbridge, Wiltshire

Contents

Acknowledgements

Sources of illustrations:
I and II, Biblioteca Nazionale Centrale, Florence; III and X, from engravings in the Library of the Royal College of Physicians, of London; IV, by gracious permission of H.M. The Queen; V, Wayland Publishers Ltd.; VI and VII, Mansell Collection; VIII and IX, The British Library; XI, Bildarchiv Preussischer Kulturbesitz, Berlin; XII, by courtesy of the Wellcome Trustees; XIII, Dr. Max Perutz. The author is indebted to the foregoing for permission to reproduce the photographs.

The author also wishes to thank Mr. L. Bradbury for supplying the quotation on p. 75, and the directors and staff of Frederick Muller Ltd., for their unfailing help and courtesy.

List of Illustrations

Introduction

Modern Views of the Heart and Blood

This introduction aims to provide the basic facts about the heart, circulation, and blood itself. It may be helpful in assessing the conclusions reached by individual pioneers. To many it will be familiar ground and they will lose nothing by proceeding straight to Chapter 1.

The heart
The heart is essentially a pump. It is divided into four chambers, two smaller thin-walled artria and two larger thicker-walled ventricles. It is composed mainly of muscle and has an outer protective layer, the pericardium. The heart muscle itself is supplied with blood by the coronary vessels.

Arteries and veins
Arteries carry blood from the heart. They have thick muscular walls to withstand the pressure of the blood pumped into them each time the heart beats. Veins return blood to the heart. The pressure of the blood in them is lower and the flow is steadier, valves at intervals preventing backflow of blood. With the exception of the pulmonary artery and pulmonary veins, blood in arteries is oxygenated and bright red in colour, blood in veins is deoxygenated and purplish red. The arteries branch repeatedly into smaller and smaller vessels, eventually becoming a network of microscopic capillaries that gradually join up again to form small veins, then larger veins.

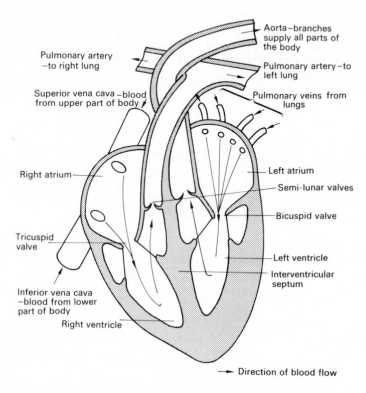

Figure 1 The heart and its associated blood vessels

The circulatory system

Man has a double circulatory system. In the lesser or pulmonary circulation, blood leaves the right ventricle of the heart in the pulmonary artery, passes through the lungs where it becomes bright red as it picks up oxygen, and returns by way of the pulmonary veins to the left atrium. It is pumped into the left ventricle, then out through the aorta on its journey round the greater or systemic circulation. During its passage all the tissues are supplied with oxygen and nutrients before the blood, now purplish red and deoxygenated, returns to the right atrium and is pumped to the right ventricle ready to set out for the lungs again.

Blood

Blood is the transport system of the body. Blood consists of red blood cells or corpuscles, white blood cells or corpuscles

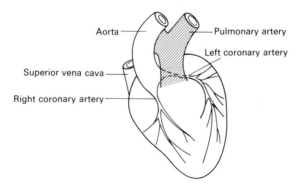

Figure 2 Coronary arteries

and platelets, all suspended in a liquid, the plasma. (Corpuscle is an older term that came into use before it was discovered that corpuscles are, in fact, cells). The red blood cells are responsible for carrying oxygen, the white blood cells are important in defending the body against infecting organisms and foreign material, and the platelets play a part in blood clotting. The plasma carries food materials, vitamins and mineral salts to the cells, and carries away carbon dioxide and other waste substances.

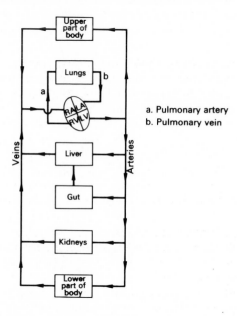

a. Pulmonary artery
b. Pulmonary vein

Figure 3 Diagram of the circulation of the blood

Chapter 1

Medicine, Magic and Religion

Prehistoric man looked upon blood with awe as it flowed from a stricken companion, wounded enemy or hunted animal. What strange properties did this red liquid possess? As many deaths occurred through injury, the sight of a body bleeding to death cannot have been unfamiliar. No wonder blood was believed to have magical properties and came to be the subject of superstition. Old Stone Age hunters, the Cro-Magnons, whose remains, dating from 20,000–8000 BC have been found in Africa and southern Europe, buried their dead with food, weapons and ornaments, and daubed the corpses or graves with blood-coloured red ochre, showing that they realised the importance of blood. Nevertheless, sometimes a man would sicken and die without losing any blood. How was this to be explained? To primitive man the environment was a source of terror with its shifting shadows and reflections, the menacing skies of an approaching storm with its attendant flashes of lightning and crashes of thunder. He attributed supernatural meanings to these phenomena, believing his world to be inhabited by spirits, demons and gods. It was all too easy to believe that demons were responsible for sickness and death, and he was only a step to convincing himself that some of his fellows were capable of magic, causing a demon to enter a man and bring about sickness. The witch doctor or medicine man was a powerful figure in the community. He combined the use of herbal remedies and other concoctions with rituals to drive the evil spirit from the sick man.

A larger-than-life figure, the medicine man often dressed in animal skins to confront the demon while he strove to banish it by suitable chants, incantations and ravings. A persistent evil spirit might be forced to depart by giving the patient a particularly nauseous concoction perhaps of animal excreta compounded with herbs. As is the nature of things, sometimes the sick man recovered, sometimes not. In such a setting the development of rational medicine, based on a knowledge of anatomy and physiology, was unlikely.

Early man was a hunter. A kill was an event of the utmost importance for it meant food for several days, but sometimes he and his companions returned empty-handed. What could be done to ensure greater success? He had already drawn larger than life-sized animals of the kind he sought, hoping to gain some power over them. What more could be done? The idea of gods was already forming in his mind, for surely some all-powerful being must ensure the sun rose every morning? Perhaps the sun itself was a god? Rain too. The grass grew lush after the rain and the animals moved on to better pasture. An offering to the gods of a portion of the next kill, or some of the animal's blood, might please the gods and make them look upon his efforts with benevolence.

In time, man discovered how to grow crops and a new and more settled way of life became possible. Offerings to the gods took the form of food and drink, newly gathered crops, a slaughtered animal or some of its blood, or in some peoples, human blood. Special ceremonies accompanied the offerings, performed by persons skilled in these matters – the priests. The roles of medicine man and priest merged. The priests became a powerful force in the community, having a direct line, as it were, to the gods. We can probably attribute to the priests the widespread belief that sickness was a punishment for sins.

In early civilisations it is not surprising to find worship of gods, witchcraft, magic and medicine closely interwoven. Any facts concerning man's beliefs about blood we can expect to find in the realms of religion as well as in medicine.

The earliest true civilisation was that of the Sumerians, a people who settled in Mesopotamia, the great alluvial plain built up by the silt of the Tigris and Euphrates rivers that flow into the Persian Gulf. The region approximates to modern Iraq.

In the fifth millenium BC, immigrant farmers came to settle in Mesopotamia. The good crops they were able to grow brought the prosperity that enabled them to leave their reed huts and simple shrines and move to mud-brick houses grouped in villages on the Tigris-Euphrates plain. The villages gave way to small towns and the early shrines to complex temples. For the first time man found that producing the basic necessities of life ceased to involve the entire community from dawn until dusk. A new factor had arisen in human affairs that was to have far-reaching consequences. It was leisure. From this small beginning, civilisations were to develop.

In the fourth millenium BC, a Central Asian people, the Sumerians, came into this productive area. The intellectual qualities and traits of character of the early settlers and the Sumerians amalgamated, and the fusion of their cultures gave rise to the earliest civilisation known, that of Sumer.

As time passed, Sumer became prosperous and politically powerful. In the city states that arose the Sumerians studied astronomy, had their own literature, religious ceremonies, code of law and doctors. They invented the wheel and the earliest form of writing known, cuneiform, a system of wedge-shaped impressions on clay. Such a thriving community was bound, sooner or later, to arouse envy, and in the third millenium BC, conquering waves of desert peoples began to surge into Mesopotamia. From Babylon the powerful King Hammurabi welded the city states into the new empire of Babylonia.

In spite of the decline in Sumerian power, life in Mesopotamia did not change greatly. However, when Hammurabi died, the empire began to disintegrate until only a small area round the capital remained. Changes were now taking place in the surrounding lands, new nations were forming and rising to power, in particular, Assyria.

In the 11th century BC, Assyria began a ruthless campaign

to conquer the Middle East. Her policy of terror and cruelty made her warriors hated and feared, but by the 7th century BC the Assyrian king, Assurbanipal, ruled over an empire extending in a vast semicircle from Egypt to the Persian Gulf. Soon a seething revolt inside Assyria augured its collapse. After a brief reflowering of Babylon under Nebuchadnessar, Babylonia was conquered by the Persian king, Cyrus. The land in which civilisation was born became part of the extensive Persian empire.

What is known about religious life and medical practice in this cauldron of Middle East civilisations? The Sumerians believed man was made from clay or clay mixed with the blood of a god. They believed that forces emanated from the gods regulating all that happened to every man, animal and plant, and therefore the only possible course was to take care to honour them. In every major city there were daily ceremonies in which food and water or wine were offered, and incense burned to please the gods. A text of the 3rd century BC contains details of the New Year festival when, following routine prayers and sacrifices, an animal was slaughtered and its bleeding body pressed against the temple walls in the belief that it absorbed all unclean elements and sins of the worshippers. It was then cast into the river. Among the gods and goddesses were a number concerned with health and sickness. Each disease was associated with a demon. Sometimes the demon himself entered the body and gave rise to the disease. Before the patient could hope to recover he had to confess his sins and the demon had to be exorcised, the assistance of the appropriate god being invoked. These activities were part of the duties of the priests who were trained in special schools and studied manuals of incantations and purification rituals. They were also concerned with divination, the art of interpreting the will of the gods and predicting future events through omens. A favourite method was to sacrifice an animal and, from the condition of the intestines or liver, read messages from the gods.

In the 19th century, archaeologists exploring featureless mounds in Mesopotamia unearthed the remains of the mud-brick city of Nippur, the religious capital of Sumer.

Large numbers of clay tablets came to light bearing pictographs and cuneiform script. One dating from 2200 BC appeared to contain a medical text. It turned out to be the oldest known manual of healing, containing a collection of prescriptions and lists of medicinal herbs together with other substances of value in medicine. It was an exciting discovery, for many of the medicinal plants such as the opium poppy, liquorice and belladonna are still in use today. Other tablets revealed the existence of a legal code on which the Law Code of Hammurabi, in the 18th century BC, was based. (A stele or a stone shaft inscribed with Hammurabi's Law Code is in the possession of the Louvre, in Paris.) Hammurabi's Code makes it clear that surgery was also being practised and laid down a scale of medical fees to be charged and the punishment to be meted out for incompetence. This shows that not only was there acquaintance with rational medical treatment but at least an elementary knowledge of anatomy.

When the Assyrians came to power in the 13th century BC, we find some modern ideas alongside directions for incantations and sacrifices. For example, they observed some connection between mosquitoes and some types of fever, and they recognised the clinical symptoms of a number of diseases including tuberculosis. A range of surgical instruments existed and one operation they are known to have performed was skull trepanning which involved the removal of a piece of bone from the skull. Such an operation may have been performed in the belief that it provided a way out for a demon who had taken possession of the body. The Assyrians were also great believers in astrology, the influence of the stars and planets on human affairs, a belief still held by some people today.

The Mesopotamian civilisation saw not only the invention of writing, but also had impressive architecture, sculpture, ornamental inlay work and beautifully carved stone cylinder seals engraved with a man's personal symbol and worn on a cord round his wrist. Their civilisation was based on a flourishing agriculture and they invented useful equipment and tools such as the seed plough and the pickaxe. They made bricks and tiles and learned to bake, sew and weave.

Goats and sheep were reared, leather tanned and made into shoes and sandals, while carpets and textiles were produced from the wool. Among the population were skilled metal-workers, glassmakers, potters, carpenters and basket-makers. The wheel was known to them and they were the first to construct an arch, building it from wedge-shaped bricks. Much was recorded on the damp clay tablets and their ideas found their way not only to neighbouring peoples but to distant lands and to communities yet unborn.

Information and ideas reached the West in several ways. When, in 586 BC, King Nebuchadnessar destroyed Jerusalem and took its people into exile in Babylon, they absorbed some of the Mesopotamian culture and learning, and when the Jews eventually returned to their homeland some of the ideas they had assimilated found their way into Christianity too, and spread with it. Even though the Mesopotamians held polytheist beliefs, their practices influenced Judaism and Christianity. A second route by which Mesopotamian culture reached the West was via Greece. The Greeks traded in the eastern Mediterranean and not only goods but ideas travelled back.

Perhaps as early as 10,000 BC man began to settle in another river valley, the fertile Nile valley, along the 1,200km stretch between the Mediterranean and the Nile cataracts, north of Khartoum. They had an advantage over the early Mesopotamians who, not being bounded by natu-ral geographical barriers, expended a great deal of energy in fighting off invaders, whereas the desert to the east and west of the Nile provided a deterrent. The scattered villages learned to co-operate in making use of the annual flooding that provided rich land for crop growing. In 3100 BC, the Egyptians were united under a ruling monarch, the first Pharaoh, who founded the city of Memphis, one of the greatest of the ancient cities. For many centuries Egypt enjoyed a stable civilisation and came to develop a remark-able culture. The river valley yielded a good crop of grain. In the delta, cattle and pigs were raised and wildfowl hunted. The Egyptians developed the art of making paper from the papyrus reeds that grew in abundance in the delta. The river provided a perfect means of communication and of transporting goods with the minimum of effort. Eventually they reached the Mediterranean and developed trade with Syria and the Lebanon, exporting grain, papyrus and linen and importing timber, copper and perfumes. The building and maintenance of the dykes was an essential activity, and was co-ordinated along the whole stretch of the river by order of the Pharaoh.

Writing dates back to the end of the fourth millenium in Mesopotamia, and the Egyptians may well have got the idea of writing from there. Both types of writing began with pictures as symbols. In Mesopotamia these soon developed into wedge-shaped strokes, but the Egyptians continued to use the small picture, the hieroglyph. The Egyptians explored engineering principles, were interested in astronomy and mathematics, and were more advanced than the Mesopotamians in medicine, but the roles of doctor and priest were still interwoven. Nevertheless, amongst the magic and incantations, wholly rational treatments evolved, particularly those dealing with physical injuries. Egyptian doctors clearly enjoyed a good reputation that extended outside their own country, for there are records of Egyptian doctors being sent to the courts of Syria, Assyria and Persia.

From their early days the ancient Egyptians had been writing down on papyrus scrolls their ideas about astronomy, stories and poems, religious and medical texts. Although the papyrus scrolls were less durable than the Mesopotamian clay tablets, the dry atmosphere of Egypt preserved them. In addition to medical papyri containing magic spells and rituals there are others with rational medical contents. One of the oldest is the Edwin Smith papyrus, discovered in a grave near Luxor, in 1862. It is believed to date from about 1600 BC and to be a copy of an older text of 3000–2500 BC. The text deals with physical injuries, wounds, fractures and dislocations, describing treatment of wounds with sutures and plasters, and methods of bone setting using splints and quick-drying resins. Clearly, the Egyptians had some knowledge of the structure of the skeleton but less about the internal organs. They realised that heart beat and pulse were in some way associated, but they knew nothing of the circulation of the blood. The text also

contains the observation that magic and medicine comple-
ment each other. If we replace the word 'magic' by 'suggestion' few modern doctors would disagree. A second
important source of information is the Ebers papyrus,
bought from an Arab in Luxor, in 1873. It was written about
1555 BC but again is a copy of older texts. It has a surgical
section, one on the heart and blood vessels, and another
on medicines. Nearly 900 medical prescriptions are noted,
and many of the ingredients, such as senna, squill and
poppy, are still in use today. Of interest is the recommen-
dation that in the treatment of certain diseases the skin
should be scratched with flint chips until blood is drawn.
Was this a forerunner of the blood letting or venesection
that gained considerable popularity much later? If so, was
it another way of ridding the body of evil spirits or their
poisons?

Early settlers in the Indus valley developed a civilisation
side by side with that of Mesopotamia and Egypt. It flour-
ished from 2500–1500 BC and occupied a far larger area than
either Egypt or Sumer. A thriving agriculture produced
wheat, barley and cotton, and well equipped ports saw the
export of gold, copper, timber, cotton and semi-precious
stones. The major fortified towns had a high standard of
hygiene, usually to be associated with good medical care.
This civilisation declined abruptly, in about 1500 BC, when
it was overrun by Aryan invaders from central Asia. The
Aryans recorded their religious beliefs and practices in four
holy books, the Vedas. The period 1500–500 BC is known as
the Vedic Age, when the fundamentals of Hinduism were
being laid down. The state of medicine in the country at the
time can be deduced from the Vedas. Intermingled with
belief in devils and magic, and the now familiar idea that
sickness was a punishment for sins, were rational methods
of healing. Knowledge of anatomy appears slight, but in
spite of this handicap there was great interest in surgery
and a firmly established belief in the purifying power of
water, a belief still to be found today. The Vedic era of
medicine persisted until about 800 BC when it was
superseded by the Brahmins, a caste of priestly wise men,
little concerned with physical illness. This proved to be an

advantage, for doctors no longer received training in temple schools, but followed an apprenticeship lasting about six years, and this essentially practical training placed medicine on a rational basis. It is clear that in the last few centuries BC, there was some exchange of ideas in medicine between India and Greece. Hippocrates, the famous Greek doctor refers to Indian drugs, and undoubtedly Alexander the Great's military expeditions to India in 327 BC and 325 BC, returned home with new ideas.

During the early centuries of the Christian era, Indian doctors began to enjoy widespread prestige. By this time, knowledge of anatomy had advanced considerably and corpses were being dissected revealing organs, muscles, blood vessels, bones and joints. Surgery was increasingly undertaken, even abdominal surgery, and there were more than a hundred surgical instruments. Over a thousand different diseases were known to these ancient doctors, and more than 700 herbs were used in healing. They suspected a connection between mosquitoes and malaria, flies and some intestinal upsets, and already they appreciated the importance of preventive medicine, including general cleanliness, suitable diet and peace of mind. They established hospitals and had a strict moral code similar to that of the Greeks.

The Middle East and India were not the only parts of the world where man was beginning to live above subsistence level and look to higher things. By 1500 BC, communities in the Yellow River valley in China were being ruled by the first king of the Shang dynasty. These people practised a simple agriculture combined with an elaborate religious and ceremonial life. The early Chinese tribes of prehistory are believed to have thought of the major features of the landscape, mountains, rivers and woods, as gods. There were also gods of natural phenomena, rain gods, wind gods and so on. Before the Shang dynasty, 1500–1000 BC, the story of Ancient China owes more to legend than to fact. The earliest rulers were given the mandate to govern by heaven, and their principal task was to communicate between the spirit world and the world of flesh and blood. The Shang kings, although no longer regarded as divine, continued to carry out the task of keeping contact with the spirit world.

The Ancient Chinese believed that when a man died his spirit went to dwell in the upper regions, where he continued to influence those he had left behind. His family brought offerings of food and wine in ritual vessels to ensure his favour. The king sought favour for his people in times of national calamity by making special offerings or sacrifices to the spirits of former kings. The spirits of former kings were nature gods or weather gods and had to be kept in benevolent moods. Regular contact had therefore to be maintained with them through a shaman, a Chinese medicine man. There are historical records of messages relayed to the royal spirits. On the death of a king, animals and servants were sacrificed, as their blood was believed to contain a spiritual power transferable to the dead monarch ensuring his future life. Blood was employed to anoint a sword, the supposed magical properties bringing success in battle. A smear of blood also confirmed the serious intent of a person taking an oath.

Reverence for and worship of ancestors was deeply rooted in Chinese tradition and was undoubtedly the reason for the taboo on the dissection of corpses. This had a far-reaching effect on Chinese medicine for it meant that knowledge of anatomy was slight. As in other early civilisations, healing and religion were closely interwoven. Priest-doctors consulted the gods about sickness, but by the 6th century BC, there were physicians distinct from priest-doctors, although they did not reject the use of charms and incantations. By the 3rd century BC, there were medical specialists who practised two forms of therapy, acupuncture and moxibustion, techniques that have their adherents in the West today. Acupuncture involves inserting special needles into the skin at specific points, while in moxibustion wicks made of wormwood (*Artemesia*) are burned and applied to the skin. An interesting text of the Han dynasty (202 BC–220 AD), called the *Huang-ti Nei Ching*, appears to contain the germ of the idea that blood circulates '. . . the river of blood traces a circle . . .'. The text is believed to be based on a much older one.

The Ancient Chinese vigorously pursued the science of astronomy, believing that knowledge of the heavens would give them power over natural phenomena. Such dangerous information, of course, had to be kept from the common people. In addition to astronomy, there was a fascination with alchemy, a belief that base metals could be turned into gold, and as gold was everlasting it became associated with immortality. Thus the search began for the elixir of life, a potion to confer immortality. As a by-product of this quest, the Chinese made important discoveries in pharmacology, the study of drugs. They found the plant *Ephedra* of value in the treatment of respiratory diseases. The active principle of the plant, ephedrine, is used today to treat asthma. Seaweed was found to be helpful in the treatment of goitre, no doubt because of the iodine content. For anaemia, fresh blood or liver was prescribed, its value only discovered in the West in the 20th century.

The Chinese made important technological advances; they invented the wheelbarrow in the 3rd century BC, and a compass during the Han dynasty; they found out how to rear silkworms and unwind the silk from cocoons and they replaced their early inscribed characters on bones by ink-brushed characters on silk scrolls, replacing the silk scrolls by paper made from rag and bark in the 2nd century AD.

During the years from 3500–2000 BC, while the civilisations of Mesopotamia, Egypt, India and China arose in the east, significant events were taking place on the other side of the world. Many thousands of years previously, before 12,000 BC, man had arrived in the New World from Asia, crossing the present Bering Strait from Siberia to Alaska. What motivated this hazardous journey across frozen tundra in such inhospitable regions? We can only guess he was seeking a better food supply or was driven out by enemies. These early immigrants spread widely in North America and lived at a very low level of subsistence. By 12,000 BC we know they were hunting big game, for beautifully made spearheads dating from this period have been found among the bones of bison and other large animals. Climatic changes, however, led to a decline in this source of food and the diet began to consist of smaller animals and more vegetable matter. Agriculture in the New World began in Mexico, the wild ancestor of maize probably grew there, and by 2500 BC early varieties of maize bearing tiny cobs helped to support a considerable population. Agricultural practice spread slowly from one suitable area to another along the mountain chain to Central and South America. By 1000 BC, agricultural communities stretched from Mexico to southern Peru, a distance of 6,400km. Crops were good and man was freed from his constant preoccupation with the seeking or producing of food. Now he had leisure, that essential prerequisite for advancement, and he began to make pottery and weave cotton cloth.

The earliest civilisation in America, dating back to 1000 BC, is that of the Olmecs. They lived in the jungles of Mexico's Gulf coast and devised a system of religious leadership that was to prove a common theme in all early American civilisations. A feature of their religion was the construction of large ceremonial centres. Olmec influence began to spread through Central America, and by the beginning of the Christian era, the impressive Teotihuacán civilisation was dawning. Between 300–700 AD, its religious centre spread to cover 18 square kilometres. It included a broad avenue, the Avenue of the Dead, a huge Pyramid of the Sun and a smaller Pyramid of the Moon. Large crowds attended the ceremonies which were conducted by priests dressed in magnificent attire who led them in their worship of the rain god, and the Feathered Serpent – a bringer of knowledge. To celebrate the coming of spring, a special ceremony involving a human sacrifice was performed.

Further south, the Maya civilisation was rising. The Mayas were great builders, their ceremonial centres being only a few kilometres apart. A small centre had a pyramid surmounted by a temple, a paved court and a number of other buildings; the larger centres had groups of pyramids with elaborately carved and brilliantly coloured temples. The Mayas devoted great energy to worshipping and placating their gods, for without their blessing who knew what disasters might befall them? The priests were exalted personages who dressed in exotic garb of coloured robes with jaguar skins and iridescent feathers of the quetzal bird, further ornamented by jade and flowers. There was an array of deities, and to propitiate them all involved almost continuous ceremonies of sacrifices and prayers. The Mayas offered sacrifices of their own blood, pricking their lips, tongue and cheeks and smearing the blood on the image of the god or on their own bodies.

In the 10th century AD, waves of barbarians from the north swept into Mexico and into the Maya centres. The religious practices of these peoples consisted of a large measure of human sacrifice. The Aztecs, whose civilisation was to be the most advanced in Ancient America, and who appeared about 1200 AD, were descendants of the barbarian tribesmen, so were the Toltecs who laid the foundations of the civilisation on which the Aztecs built. The Toltecs originated the belief that the sun fought a daily battle with the night and needed nourishment of warm blood and human hearts, or next day it might be too weak to rise, darkness would spread over the land and all life would perish.

The Aztecs founded the city of Tenochtitlán which later became Mexico City. There were other cities in the Valley of Mexico, but the Aztecs rose to power by craftily setting one against the other. They were a warring people who worshipped Huitzilopochtli, the 'hummingbird-on-the-left-hand', their war and sun god, who led their warriors in battle and, according to their beliefs, watched over them. They exploited their defeated enemies ruthlessly. The captives they took were sacrificed to Huitzilopochtli, while from the conquered people they demanded reparations in the form of weapons and essential supplies for their own warriors. Their increasingly well-equipped army went on to gain further victories and the grateful Aztecs were able to sacrifice even more victims to Huitzilopochtli. The human sacrifices amounted almost to an industry. In the city stood the temple pyramid and other grand buildings, presided over by the priests who mounted the steps of the pyramid carrying burning incense to please the gods. Within the temple, black-robed priests led each victim to the sacrificial stone where he was flung on his back, some priests holding him down by his arms and legs while another priest carved into the man's chest with a sharp obsidian knife cutting out and holding up the still beating heart. When the temple was dedicated to Huitzilopochtli, more than 20,000 captives were sacrificed. Their beliefs led them to accept that it was an honour to be sacrificed, an honour equal to that of death in battle, in either case they would be assured of a glorious afterlife. The dedication ceremonies lasted several days, the long queue of victims moving slowly forward towards the sacrificial stone, where pools of blood formed as the pile of corpses grew. Civilians too, had their role to play, they could offer blood from self-inflicted wounds to the God of the Dead. There was another side to Aztec life, however, an enjoyment of feasts and festivals with music, dancing and flowers, in honour of the lesser gods.

In the Inca civilisation that arose in Peru about 1200 AD, religious ceremonies never played such a prominent role. Human sacrifice was reserved for times of great emergency.

In 1521, the Aztec kingdom fell to the Spaniard, Cortés, and was brought under the rule of the Spanish crown, the inhuman practices of the Aztecs providing a convenient excuse for the take-over. To the astonishment of the Spaniards they found that the Aztecs had a higher standard of hygiene than was to be found in many European cities, and, moreover, their medical practice proved to be well developed. There were well stocked pharmacies, the Aztecs making use of over a thousand plants for medicinal purposes. They set broken bones, even plating fractures, performed Caesarean sections, and sewed up wounds with human hair. Ten years later, in 1531, another Spaniard, Pizarro, conquered the Inca empire in Peru. Although the Incas worshipped a number of gods and believed that the cause of illness lay in the sins of the patient, they had a medical system superior to the Aztecs in surgery. They removed tumours, carried out amputations and trepanning. Annually they held a health festival in which all houses and public buildings were thoroughly cleaned.

Chapter 2

The Greeks Develop Rational Medicine

In the third millenium BC, people surged into the Greek peninsular from the north, filtering gradually south and being obliged to settle in small groups owing to the mountainous nature of the country. Although the groups had little communication with each other they were basically one people, speaking dialects of the same language, worshipping the same gods and, in time, developing their city states on similar lines. As few inhabitants were out of sight of the sea they became able mariners. On trading forays they made full use of the many scattered islands in the Mediterranean as stepping stones to the establishment of colonies from Spain to the Black Sea. The city state was a mixed blessing for, on the one hand, much energy was wasted in feuds between the city states, but on the other, not being subjected to an all powerful central control, the individual had opportunities for the development of self reliance and personal freedom. Athens became the leading city state, a centre of cultural and intellectual life, but in time internal discord led to the attentions of King Philip of Macedonia who became the ruler of Greece in 338 BC. His son, Alexander the Great was to extend the Greek empire as far as India.

The Greeks were favourably located to receive the stimulus of ideas and influences from the civilisations of Egypt and Mesopotamia, and also from India through the military expeditions of Alexander the Great. These new ideas were absorbed by a people who believed in the freedom of the individual to develop his own potential to the full. No inflexible theology hampered the Greeks in their desire for knowledge, for although they believed in a plethora of gods, acknowledging them to be the source of their own physical and mental abilities, they believed it to be their personal responsibility to develop these gifts to the full, thus art, science and religion existed happily side by side. The offering of prayers and sacrifices to the gods and the consulting of oracles in no way conflicted with their search for truth.

In the past there had been occasional glimpses of rational medicine, but it was the Ancient Greeks who developed a medical science independent of religion and magic, although parallel with it there survived a belief in the healing power of the god, Asclepios. He was believed to perform miracles, even raising the dead. Shrines were erected in his honour, the most famous being Epidaurus in the Peloponnese, which became a place of pilgrimage and a health resort. The Romans later adopted Asclepios, (to them he was Aesculapius), and he was depicted holding a staff with an entwined snake, the staff was a feature of the travelling physician and the snake a symbol of renewal, owing to its habit of sloughing off the skin to reveal a new one underneath. The snake twined round a staff has remained a symbol of medicine ever since.

In the 6th century BC, a Greek doctor, Alcmaeon of Croton, born about 500 BC, on the Gulf of Taranto, was one of the first to practise animal dissection. Animals at this time would be killed by bleeding and this fact, or an early confusion between blood vessels and air tubes, probably accounts for a statement in Alcmaeon's textbook that there were two types of blood vessel, one empty after death. Alcmaeon believed, with remarkable perception for his time, that the brain was the site of mental activity.

On the beautiful island of Cos, in the Aegean Sea, lived the most famous doctor of all time, Hippocrates. Born about 460 BC, he was revered in his lifetime, and honoured in the Middle Ages by the title of 'Father of Medicine', for, at that time, nothing was known of medicine from pre-Greek civilisations. The professional skill and compassion of Hippocrates made him the leading doctor in Greece and he is said to have travelled extensively, even being called to the courts of the kings of Macedonia and Persia. Hippocrates is said to have gathered around him a group of physicians who believed in the medical principles he advocated, and thus they formed an early school of medicine. A number of generations of doctors who were followers of Hippocrates probably contributed to the 72 books known as the *Corpus Hippocraticus* (Hippocratic Collection), brought to Alexandria in the 3rd century BC. Some of the works were intended for medical students, others for the public; among them are lectures to students, research and clinical notes, philosophical essays, and books on air, water, places, diet, epidemics, and treatment of acute diseases. One, *About the Nature of Man*, describes a theory of humours or body liquids, lack of balance between them supposedly giving rise to illness.

Hippocrates concerned himself with the whole patient. He used few medicines considering it wiser to discover what Nature was trying to do, and refrained from interfering with natural healing processes. Instead he supported these processes by means of rest, fresh air, cleanliness and a good diet. Excellent advice considering the limited knowledge of anatomy and physiology at the time, and advice that can be overlooked in these days of sophisticated medication. By his rational approach, Hippocrates placed medicine on a scientific basis, and once freed from the cloud of myth, magic and superstition as well as the idea that sickness was a punishment for sins, the way was clear for others to follow. One of the great contributions Hippocrates made was his formulation and teaching of the rules of conduct to be observed by doctors. These are incorporated in the Hippocratic oath, still taken in a similar form today by medical students on qualifying: 'Into whatsoever houses I enter, I will enter to help the sick, and I will abstain from all intentional wrongdoing and harm . . . and whatsoever I shall see or hear . . . if it be what should not be published abroad, I will never divulge.'

Did Hippocrates make any great discoveries about the blood system? Not as far as we know, but he certainly carried out dissections and decided that blood vessels were of two distinct types. He also believed that blood travelled from the liver and spleen to be warmed by the heart.

In 377 BC, the greatest of the Greek philosophers and one of the most universally respected of learned men was born in Stagira, in Macedonia. His name was Aristotle and he lived from 384–322 BC. He came from a family with a medical background; his father was physician to the King and all his brothers were doctors. As a young man Aristotle, who was of phenomenal intellect, moved to Athens, having been attracted by the cultural and intellectual life centred there. He attended lectures given by the great philosopher, Plato, and became his star pupil. After Plato died in 347 BC, Aristotle went to Mytilene on the island of Lesbos where for the next two years he delighted in biological studies that had a profound influence on the nature of his philosophy. In 342 BC, he was summoned to the court of King Philip who required him to tutor his son, Alexander. Six years passed, the King was assassinated, and his son, who was to become the famous soldier Alexander the Great, succeeded him. Aristotle returned to Athens where he founded the Lyceum, educating most of the leading intellectuals of his day. Aristotle's lectures were collected into 400 volumes. They laid the foundations for the study of science, logic, ethics, political thought and literature, and came to be revered as indisputable authority until the 17th century.

Aristotle, whose teaching was far in advance of his time, believed that true knowledge was based on observation and experience. In his pursuit of knowledge of anatomy, he was restricted by the prevailing objections to dissection of the human body, but he was a pioneer in the dissection of animals. In place of bleeding he introduced strangulation of the animals, but unfortunately, from the point of view of gaining information about the heart and blood vessels, this method resulted in congestion on the venous side of the heart. This led Aristotle to mistake the right atrium together with the right ventricle for a single chamber, even though he distinguished the atrium from the ventricle on the left side, so that he came to the conclusion that the heart was three chambered. Strangulation also left the arteries empty of blood and Aristotle made no clear distinction between them and veins, although he was aware of the connection between the heart and the blood vessels. Aristotle believed that the heart, not the brain, was the centre of physical and mental processes, a belief that survived long after the discovery of the controlling influence of the brain. Today, over 2,300 years later, the idea persists in everyday speech, for example, 'heartache' indicates an emotional experience rather than a physical pain, and we may use 'lion-hearted' as a synonym for brave.

During the 13 years of his reign, Alexander the Great conquered the extensive Persian Empire spreading Greek culture through an area fifty times larger than Greece itself. He founded many cities, including Alexandria, named after him. On his death, in 323 BC, one of his generals, Soter, declared himself King of Egypt. He became Ptolemy 1. During his reign a well-equipped medical school and an extensive library of papyrus scrolls were founded in Alexandria, attracting two leading Greek teachers in the early days, Herophilus of Chalcedon (333–280 BC), and Erasistratus of Chios (310–250 BC). They were able to establish the practice of dissection of the human body, there being little opposition from the Egyptians at that time owing to their own custom of embalming the dead.

Herophilus, undeterred by the reverence accorded to the teachings of Aristotle, declared that the brain was the controlling organ of the body. He demonstrated that arteries had thicker walls than veins and he named the thick-walled vessel leading from the right ventricle to the lungs (pulmonary artery), the artery-like vein, presumably because it was found to contain dark venous blood. The thin-walled vessels leading from the lungs to the left atrium (pulmonary veins), he named the vein-like arteries, probably finding them to contain bright red blood. He was convinced that the heart sent blood to the arteries and he appreciated that the function of the lungs was to take in fresh air, distribute it, and collect and expel stale air.

Erasistratus examined the heart and deduced that the bicuspid and tricuspid valves and the semi-lunar valves functioned to allow materials to pass in one direction only. He came to the conclusion that blood was pumped through the heart on the right side, but he thought air reached the left side of the heart from the lungs and was carried round the body in the arteries, this air he called 'vital spirit'. In spite of the fact that the arteries could be found to contain blood, Erasistratus maintained this only happened at death or when the body was diseased or injured, a view that continued to be upheld for over 400 years. Although Erasistratus was off the rails in his views about the circulatory system, he pointed out that the highly convoluted cerebrum in the human brain was related to man's superior intelligence, and he agreed with Herophilus that the brain was the controlling organ.

Herophilus and Erasistratus made the medical school of Alexandria famous. It remained the leading centre of learning in the medical sciences for 200 years, until Caesar came on the scene. When Caesar conquered Egypt and assimilated it into the Roman Empire, Rome itself became the new centre giving us the next landmarks in our story.

Chapter 3

Galen of Pergamum, a Greek in Rome

There was a very famous doctor in Imperial Rome in the 2nd century AD, who was a Greek by birth, and whose name was Galen (130–200 AD). He was born in Pergamum, in Asia Minor, a city that once contained a shrine to the god of healing, Asclepios, as well as an extensive library. Galen studied at the school of philosophy in his home city, and in his late teens he received tuition from the doctor, Satyros, a specialist in anatomy and author of a learned textbook on the subject. After the death of his father, Galen became restless and made up his mind to travel. He first visited Smyrna and Corinth, but the idea of going to Alexandria, still a famous centre of learning and research, grew in his mind. Alexandria was everything he had dreamed about; it continued to enjoy the fine reputation that had begun in the days of Herophilus and Erastistratus, and it was, he believed, a place where knowledge could be pursued in a true spirit of freedom. In actual fact it was less free than in former days, for now that it was under the control of Rome, human dissection was forbidden. Nevertheless, Galen gained considerable knowledge of anatomy by dissecting the bodies of animals.

When Galen was about 30 years of age, he went back to Pergamum to practise as a doctor. He was appointed to attend the wounded gladiators during the festivals, and thus earned a reputation for his skill in the treatment of wounds which aided him in building a successful private practice. After four years of this he looked around for further challenges. Where was he to go? Why not the Imperial metropolis, Rome? But whereas in Pergamum he had been a person of some importance, in Rome he was unknown – but not for long. He was called to attend a celebrated philosopher who was suffering from malaria; the patient had already been attended by other doctors who had failed to bring him relief, but Galen was able to cure him. Galen's name soon reached the ears of leading families in the city and he found himself much in demand, and being very well rewarded financially. He was able to continue with his research through a contact at the court, himself interested in anatomy, who obtained animals for the two men to dissect together. After four years, Galen returned to Pergamum. We don't know why. Perhaps he had tired of Rome or of the jealousy he had aroused in other doctors by his greater success, or perhaps he yearned for a sight of his native city. On the other hand, he may have travelled back to escape an epidemic of smallpox that was sweeping through Rome. Whatever it was, before long the Emperor, Marcus Aurelius, recalled him to Rome and Galen soon found he had a very busy life again. In addition to being the Emperor's personal physician, he attended his patients, lectured, researched and made time to write on medical topics and logic. He remained in Rome for the next thirty years.

Galen believed there must be a connection between the structure of an organ, its purpose and its method of functioning. He drew heavily on the authorities of his day and wrote a book on the uses of the organs that remained a standard work for 1,400 years. His researches into the nervous system showed the difference between cranial and spinal nerves, but he thought they were hollow and carried 'psychic' or 'animal spirit' from the ventricles in the brain. He demonstrated that arteries were filled with blood and not air as Herophilus and Erastistratus had taught. One experiment Galen conducted was to tie an artery of a living animal in two places and show that the isolated length contained blood. He believed in the accepted teaching that air had to be distributed round the body to keep it alive, but as the arteries had been believed to contain air, they were thought to be responsible for distributing it. Now, he reasoned, having shown that arteries contain blood, blood in the arteries must take the air round the body. The question was, how did air get into the blood? First of all, he believed, food was absorbed in the stomach and transported to the liver where blood was continuously manufactured and where 'natural spirit' also arose. Veins from the liver distributed blood for nourishment through the body, and some entered the right ventricle of the heart (Galen ignored the atria). On inspiration, he reasoned, air filled the lungs and as the heart expanded (diastole), air passed down the venous arteries (pulmonary veins) to the left ventricle of the heart where it combined with blood passing through invisible pores in the interventricular septum from the right ventricle, changing in colour from purplish-red to bright red. In this process, he thought, 'vital spirit' was made. The blood was then sucked out by the pulsation of the arteries and distributed to the tissues. According to Galen's views, every tissue received 'natural spirit' from the veins, 'vital spirit' from the arteries and 'psychic' or 'animal spirit' from the nerves.

Galen was a good doctor who believed, unlike Hippocrates, that illness was of local origin. He was less inclined to let Nature take its course, but prescribed bleeding, purging and complex formulations of herbs. Even today prescriptions with many ingredients are known as 'Galenic' preparations. In spite of his pirating of the views of others and his apparent lack of humility, Galen was a great experimentalist who made a considerable contribution to the study of anatomy. As Roman regulations forbade dissection of the human body, he studied in detail the anatomy of different kinds of animals, but unfortunately he applied what he learned to the human body. Such was his excellent reputation as a doctor that his pronouncements were accepted without question, facts and errors alike. In scientific research, an erroneous statement or false conclusion is usually soon challenged by others, but in that particular climate, no one considered challenging the opinions of the great Galen. Nor, as it turned out, were they seriously challenged for over a thousand years. Galen's death marked the end of an era in scientific research, for the impetus in the search for knowledge that had developed in Classical Greece, waned in the Roman Empire. The seeds of decline were already sown when Galen died in 200 AD. Medical science slowly withered during the unsettled times that followed, several factors contributing to its demise. Firstly, a catastrophic malaria epidemic swept through the Roman Empire in the 3rd century; secondly, the new religion of Christianity proved to be suspicious of scientists and philosophers, although the established views of the learned Greek, Galen, were deemed to be respectable. Then, invasions by the Goths, Huns and Vandals began which culminated in the fall of Rome in 410 AD. With Rome gone, the western Roman Empire quickly followed leaving Byzantium as the capital of the Empire. By then, Galen's views were firmly entrenched, and were to remain so throughout the Middle Ages when unquestioning faith in authority was expected. To question Galen's teaching was regarded as heresy.

Chapter 4

The Middle Ages

In the 5th century AD, in the hot dry land of Arabia, there dwelt nomadic Bedouin tribesmen surviving on a meagre diet of milk and dates and living in tents of goat and camel hair. They were united by the necessity born of a harsh environment in which each man was in need of the support of his neighbour. By the middle of the 6th century, towns were appearing in the north, the largest being Mecca. Situated on the crossroads of two important caravan routes, it was the site of Arabia's most important pagan shrine. Here several hundred gods were worshipped, the most important being Allah, the Creator of the Universe.

In the year 570 AD, the Prophet Mohammed was born in Mecca. The small religious community he later collected around him grew into the mighty empire of Islam. It was to have a profound influence upon the world. As a young adult, Mohammed worked as a shepherd, then as a trader, before he took a job with the wealthy widow, Khadija. This involved him in travelling north to Syria on her behalf, where he met many Jews and Christians. He was impressed by their firm beliefs and fell to reflecting upon the need for a unifying faith among his own people. He married Khadija who bore his seven children. His marriage freed him from poverty and gave him time for meditation. When he reached the age of 40, a mystical event occurred in his life, it was revealed to him that he was to become an apostle of God. Mohammed was troubled by this but at the end of a further three years he had a second vision in which he was commanded to commence work. In Mecca, in 613 AD, he began teaching that Allah was the one true God and that all believers were equal before him. In the next few years, he and his followers met with fierce opposition which led them to move to Medina in 622 AD. This was the dawn of Islam. Mohammed's following grew, and by the time he died, in 632 AD, at the age of 62, he had built up a belief in a single god, fused it to a fierce Arab nationalism that had lain dormant, and left his people with a cause for which they could unite and fight. Within the next century, Islam's fervent forces swept out of Arabia, through Asia, Africa and into Europe, establishing a vast empire exceeding that of the Romans. For 600 years Islamic religion and culture were dominant. Egyptians, Turks, Persians, Indians, Africans and Spaniards were linked by the Koran, a collection of Mohammed's oral revelations, and as a translation of the Koran was forbidden, they were also united by the Arabic language.

After the death of Mohammed, Islam was ruled by a succession of Caliphs. A new capital was founded in Damascus where a distinct Islamic culture began to evolve; lavish palaces were built for the Caliphs, public works were undertaken and beautiful mosques constructed. The most famous Caliph was Harun al-Rashid (786–809 AD), of *The Arabian Nights* fame, who made a new capital at the important trade centre of Baghdad. Baghdad in those days was the major trading centre of the world and it came to reflect the growing Persian influence. From Islam's extensive empire, caravans and ships brought grain and fruits, rich silks and linen, precious metals and gem stones, porcelain and exotic perfumes. With them came something of even greater value – new ideas. Dormant in Islam lay the culture left by the Greeks and the time was now ripe for its re-awakening.

Islam began to look at the world from a new point of view, basically the point of view of Classical Greece: that fundamentally the world was an orderly place and with questioning and reasoning, its laws might be discovered. This new outlook fused with ideas from Persia and India, and produced an upsurge of interest in science, philosophy, theology and literature. The famous Greek library in Alexandria had been destroyed by the Romans in the 1st century AD, but records of the work of the Ancient Greek scientists and philosophers still survived elsewhere. The works of famous Greeks such as Aristotle, Plato, Ptolemy, Hippocrates and Galen, were sought out and translated into Arabic. An eminent scholar, responsible for translating Galen's works, was Hunayn ibn Ishaq, who had studied medicine under a doctor trained in the famous Persian medical school of Gondeshapur; having added Greek to his accomplishments, he showed not only skill in translation but developed a talent for seeking out Greek manuscripts. In time he was appointed assistant physician to the Caliph and eventually came to be in charge of translations in the House of Wisdom, the centre of learning in Baghdad. He wrote a number of medical books of his own, including a treatise on ophthalmology, thus he helped to lay the foundations of modern medicine, for, in time, his work was translated into Latin and found its way to the West.

To the House of Wisdom, in the 9th century, came scientists, artists, philosophers, theologians and poets. There was an instinctive understanding that a wide spectrum of knowledge, rather than a narrow specialisation, would lead to the solving of some of the mysteries of the world. Thus there arose the scientist-philosopher, a man of wide learning in many branches of science; medicine, chemistry, astronomy and mathematics, as well as in philosophy and perhaps music and literature too. Few, of course, were of this stature and in order to be free to pursue knowledge for its own sake they needed a rich patron to support them. Such patrons were forthcoming, enabling the fame of Baghdad to grow, drawing students from all quarters of the Empire. Although knowledge was sought primarily for its own sake, Islam did not neglect the possible practical applications of new discoveries.

When some of the old Greek medical prescriptions and treatments had been translated, Islam used and developed them for use in place of the charms and folk remedies that had been used before. In the 9th and 10th centuries most of the doctors were of Persian origin, although they spoke

Arabic which was the language of the educated man of the time. Many had received their training at Gondeshapur, where Hunayn ibn Ishaq had studied. One of the best known was Zakkariya al-Razi (860–930 AD), better known by the Latin version of his name, Rhazes. Rhazes was senior physician at Baghdad's largest hospital and was responsible for laying down rules of hygiene far in advance of his time. He was also a talented chemist who recorded his experiments in such detail that they can be repeated today. As the result of one experiment he made plaster of Paris and was quick to see how useful it would be to hold broken bones in place. He wrote a large number of books and compiled an encyclopaedia, *El Hawl*, of Greek, Syrian, Persian, Indian and Arabic medical knowledge, adding many of his own observations and conclusions – it was to have a wide influence in the West later.

Half a century after Rhazes died, an even more famous Arabic-speaking Persian doctor was born, his name was Abdullah Ibn Sina (980–1037 AD), known to the West as Avicenna. Avicenna was a child prodigy who readily absorbed any knowledge offered him. He wrote books on medicine, philosophy, astronomy, mathematics and theology, and also composed poems. Although he was self taught in medicine he compiled an encyclopaedia, containing much of his own work, called *The Canon of Medicine*. It was outstandingly successful and became the standard textbook in the East for many centuries. It was later translated into Latin and in time became the most frequently printed work.

In the 12th and 13th centuries, two of the most famous hospitals were those in Damascus and Cairo. There was close co-operation between Egypt and Syria in the field of medicine, and at one time they shared an official who supervised medical care. His name was Al-Dakhwar. One of his most important supporters was Ibn al-Nafis, philosopher, theologian and physician, who had studied medicine in Damascus and had afterwards taken up an appointment as chief physician at the Nasiri Hospital, in Cairo. He was also personal physician to the Marmaluke ruler, Beibars Bandukdary, who reigned from 1260 to 1277. In addition to medical work, Ibn al-Nafis lectured in jurisprudence in Cairo and was an authority on religious law. He was a prolific writer. While only in his early thirties he wrote *A Comprehensive Book on the Art of Medicine*, believed to consist of 300 volumes of notes on medicine and surgery, of which 80 were published. In 1952, an exciting discovery was made: one volume was found among the Cambridge University Library's Islamic manuscripts. This led to the discovery that many years before, four manuscripts had been catalogued at the Bodleian Library, Oxford, the author at that time being unidentified. In 1960, three more manuscripts were found in the medical library of Stanford University, USA.

Ibn al-Nafis wrote a commentary on the work of Hippocrates, the Greek physician, a volume on eye diseases (a speciality of Islamic physicians), and volumes on logic and theology, in addition to his reference work for physicians. From our point of view, his most interesting work was *Commentary on Anatomy in Books 1 and 111 of Ibn Sina's Canon of Medicine*. In this *Commentary* is to be found the earliest known account of the lesser or pulmonary circulation of the blood. Ibn al-Nafis went on to write *Commentary upon the Canon*, a four-volume work. In Volume 1, he again gives his theory of the pulmonary circulation. Concerning the ventricles he states categorically, 'there is no passage between these two cavities which would allow passage of blood, as Galen thought'. Although he uses names for the pulmonary artery and pulmonary veins that are not used today, it is quite clear that he is referring to these vessels and that he appreciates that blood must pass from the right ventricle to the left ventricle by way of the lungs. Authorities have put the date of his discovery around 1242.

Ibn al-Nafis tells us his religion prevented him from carrying out anatomical research. He makes it clear, however, that in giving his opinion he relied on personal examination and research, taking no heed of whether or not his opinion agreed or disagreed with those who had gone before. In the religious climate of the time, dissection of the human body would have been regarded as an act of desecration performed on God's supreme creation, and in any case Islamic law did not permit it. Now, Ibn al-Nafis was both physician and theologian as well as an authority on religious law. Do we assume, in this case, his research took the form of exercise of his very able intelligence? This is not the end of the story of Ibn al-Nafis, but to tell it now would be to anticipate events. We shall return to him in a later chapter.

From the 9th to the 14th century, Islam kept the disciplines of Greek science alive, adding to it valuable discoveries of its own. Medicine found Islam a more convenient place for its development than the West under the domination of the Christian church.

In the West in the 11th and 12th centuries, there was a revival of interest in the sciences, due in some measure to the work of Constantine the African (Constantinius Africanus). He was born in North Africa in 1020 AD, and spent many years travelling for the purpose of studying oriental languages, and the medical practices and philosophies of the ancient civilisations. In later life he became a monk and passed the rest of his days in the monastery of Monte Cassino, between Rome and Naples, where he carefully and systematically translated the ancient classical medical literature from Arabic into Latin. (The monastery was severely damaged in the 1939–45 war. It has been restored and the chapel is being enriched with frescoes by the world-famous artist Pietro Annigoni, who is carrying out the work as a labour of love.) Before the turn of the 12th century, Constantine had translated Galen's *Art of Medicine and Therapeutics*, as well as an Arabic treatise on ophthalmology. Thus, Greek medical science, after a long journey from Rome to Constantinople and eastwards to Persia, returned to Italy many centuries later. Soil favourable for its growth was waiting.

The famous medieval medical school of Salerno began life in a pilgrim hospital annexed to a monastery. The school was founded by laymen and consequently it was able to throw off the controlling hand of the Church. It was open to all, men and women alike, of any nationality, educating them in the newly rediscovered medical science. Salerno not only served as a model for the major universities yet to be established, but it was instrumental in bringing into force legislation allowing only those with proper medical training to practise. By the end of the 12th century, other medical schools in Paris, Bologna, Oxford and Montpellier had been established, to be followed by those of Naples, Messina and Padua. Their professors of medical science were clergymen, so the new courses were tailored to some extent to fit the views of the Church. In 1163, the Synod of Tours had proclaimed, *Ecclesia abhorret a sanguine* (The Church abhors bloodshed), by and large, therefore, doctors ceased to practise surgery and it fell into the hands of barbers and quacks. Nevertheless, with a number of centres providing a systematic medical training, some educated minds began to question the views of Galen and soon found themselves in conflict with the Church. It was a dangerous time to hold original ideas and to express them was to invite the attention of the Inquisition (A body of Cardinals who tried people for disseminating views not in accordance with orthodox religious teaching).

In England, Roger Bacon (1214–94) physician, philosopher and scientist, was urging scholars to lay aside the works of the Ancients and study anew the wonders of nature. Bacon had studied in Oxford and Paris and had become a Franciscan friar. He was able to read both Arabic and Greek and was convinced that there was no way forward except by direct personal observation and practical experiment. He, himself, dissected animals and probably human corpses too. (How else could he have become familiar with the structure of the human brain and eye?) He was a man far in advance of his time, prophesying the invention of horseless carriages, fast boats, and machines in which man would conquer the skies like a bird. He was soon ordered to stop writing and teaching such revolutionary notions, but he enjoyed a brief respite when Pope Clement IV (1265–68) commanded him to set down his views. This Bacon did, in three major works. The death of Pope Clement brought this support to an end, and he was cast into prison for his heretical views and only released after 14 years, two years before he died. His words, however, echoed down the years and were heard by others born in more propitious times.

Roger Bacon's advanced ideas seem the more remarkable if we look briefly at the social conditions and the standard of care of the sick in England in the half millenium before Bacon's birth. It was a time of malnutrition and low standards of hygiene, encouraging lice, fleas and larger vermin that in their turn assisted epidemic diseases to sweep through the land. Strange pagan ideas were widespread among the people; they believed in supernatural creatures of the forests and moorland, and in elves that threw darts at them, the 'elfshot' producing pain and disease. They put their faith in charms and in herbs, not solely as remedies but as a protection against evil.

To the Anglo-Saxons the doctor was known as the leech (the Old English word is *laece*). He knew little about specific diseases or about anatomy and physiology, the works of Hippocrates and Galen lay largely forgotten, he relied on folk remedies, his treatments consisting of diets together with herbal and animal materials used in the form of ointments, powders, poultices, lotions or draughts. Incantations and charms were as much part of his stock-in-trade as the preparations themselves. Incantations might be employed during the gathering of the ingredients, preparation of the remedy or over the sick patient. Exorcisms were practised to expel evil spirits or attempts made to transfer the disease from the patient to some object, by means of rites and ceremonies. Beads and certain plants were believed to afford protection from disease, and teeth or shells were commonly employed in the belief that childbirth would be eased.

A common practice in Anglo-Saxon England, and one already well established in the 7th century, was bloodletting or venesection. Apart from a possible belief that venesection let evil spirits out of the body, one reason for the practice was the conviction that too much blood was a cause of illness. (Did this conviction arise through some half-forgotten view held by Galen that blood was being made continuously in the liver?) The site chosen for the opening of a vein was related to the type of illness, and the day and time were chosen with due regard to the season of the year, phases of the moon and astrological considerations. To fail to take account of seasonal and cosmic matters was considered to invite disaster. Blood-letting was commonly practised in the monasteries as a prophylactic as well as a curative measure. At such a time, a monk would enjoy some relaxation of rules, small comforts and a more nourishing diet. Obtaining permission to be bled came to be abused as a means of having a change from the rigorous routine and frugal meals. The practice of blood-letting was not without its dangers, uncontrollable bleeding and sepsis being two not uncommon complications. Scarification, superficial cutting or scratching of the skin was sometimes employed as an alternative to blood-letting, and it might be combined with cupping, a practice of applying a cup-like vessel which had been warmed, over the skin to draw the blood to the area as it cooled. Blood-letting and cupping survived into modern times.

In England, true leprosy first made its appearance in the 7th century, reaching its peak in the 12th century and then declining, probably as a result of some improvement in diet and living conditions. Various tests were made to diagnose the disease and distinguish it from other skin ailments. One relied on certain supposed properties of the blood, it was thought that the blood of a leper was thicker and clotted more rapidly than normal blood and that a drop added to water would float on the surface whereas a drop of normal blood would sink. One sensible treatment prescribed the eating of only fresh food, adding a cautious note to avoid food 'that overheats the blood'. Blood-letting would be carried out if the patient was strong enough.

Half a century after Roger Bacon died in 1294, plague reached the Crimea from the east and swept like a flame across Europe. This deadly epidemic, marking the end of the Middle Ages, became known as the Black Death. It killed 25 million people in Europe, a quarter of the population.

Chapter 5

The Science of Human Anatomy is Born

The terrible plague of the 14th century faded away. In Italy the growing trade of the city republics was giving rise to a new wealthy and powerful ruling class whose leisure and means gave them a taste for cultural pursuits. From them and through their patronage of the arts there came a revival of interest in Greek and Roman culture that led not only to the development of a new, vigorous and less formal style in all branches of the arts, but to a new intellectual awakening. People began to question established authority in all walks of life, and there was a growing desire for individuality and self expression. The re-awakening or rebirth was the Renaissance. There was a great flourishing of talent, among the greatest the names of Leonardo de'Luzzi, Michelangelo and Raphael stand out. From Italy the new ideas spread gradually over Western Europe assisted by the development of printing.

Poised on the threshold of this new period, and very much part of it, intellectually, was Mondino de'Luzzi, or Mondinus (1275–1326). He studied medicine at the University of Bologna, and taught anatomy there from about 1306. Dissection of human cadavers, previously banned, was re-introduced primarily for legal reasons, to investigate the cause of death under suspicious circumstances. It led to demonstration dissections for the benefit of students, to enable them to become familiar with the teachings of Galen, on anatomy. Mondino broke away from the established practice of lecturing from a high platform while an assistant carried out the dissection below; instead he performed the dissection himself, and in the process, discovered certain details at variance with the authority of Galen. In 1315, he published a book on anatomy that contained much traditional material together with new facts, the result of his own observations – it was not to be superseded until the time of Vesalius, 200 years later. Mondino's successors, who perhaps preferred to keep their distance from the often far-from-fresh corpse, abandoned the practice of performing their own dissections and reverted to the earlier system.

In the mid-15th century, one of the most outstanding men of all time was born – Leonardo da Vinci (1452–1519). Not only was he a superlative artist but he held theories about engineering and dynamics centuries ahead of his time. Ranking with his ability as an artist, were his skills as inventor and scientist. He insisted on the need for experiment, recording his ideas, observations and comments in voluminous notebooks, writing with his left hand from right to left forming 'mirror writing'. Scholars have found a full evaluation of Leonardo's work to be a difficult task for a number of reasons: some of his notebooks and papers were lost (they are turning up even now – the latest find was a notebook discovered in Madrid and published in 1974), his notes were in great confusion, they are difficult to read and sometimes not easy to interpret, with their abbreviations, ideas in the form of sketches and a mixture of topics on the same page. As his ideas developed, he might return again and again to the same subject, sometimes noting down contradictory statements but leaving no clue about the order in which he formed his ideas. A stream of original thoughts poured from his versatile mind and it is probable that he never organised himself sufficiently well to prepare his work for publication, although in an uncompleted will he urged his successors to do so. When he died he left his notebooks and drawings to his young friend and pupil, Francesco Melzi (1491–1568), who collected together all the notes he could find on painting and published *The Treatise on Painting* under Leonardo's name, in 1651. He also carried out considerable cataloguing, but after his death the papers became dispersed.

At the time of Leonardo's birth, Italy was divided into five independent states, Florence, Milan, Venice, Rome and Naples, each ruled by a dictator who relied on mercenaries or intrigue to maintain his position and keep his boundaries intact. Leonardo was born in Vinci, near Florence, and was apprenticed to the artist Verrochio, becoming a member of the painters' guild at the age of 20. His biographer, Vasari, describes him as having a 'lavish abundance' of 'beauty, grace and ability'. With his outstanding artistic and engineering abilities he did not want for patrons, and he spent most of his life in the employ of rulers who made use of his engineering skills to defend their states and his artistic talent to enhance their prestige. He worked in Florence under the patronage of Lorenzo the Magnificent of the House of Medici, and later in Milan in the service of Ludovico Sforza. For a short time Cesare Borgia, son of Pope Alexander VI, was his patron, and he spent his last years in the employ of Francis 1, of France. All the while Leonardo was working on his artistic commissions and engineering projects he was pursuing his scientific enquiries and developing his numerous inventions. During his lifetime he invented over 400 devices including a water mill, paddle wheel, crane, shearing machine and dredger. He studied bird flight in order to design flying machines, and the movement of fish with plans for a submarine in mind. He invented machinery to make tools for his work, treadle-operated lathes, mechanical saws and boring equipment, and later he built his own copies of clocks, compasses and other instruments for his scientific work. He made extensive investigations in anatomy – sheets of meticulous drawings and notes on human and animal anatomy survive.

Leonardo began his investigations into anatomy by studying the standard textbooks of the time that were of Galenic or Arabic origin, and he set out with humility to discover the structures noted by his distinguished predecessors. Only when he found his own observations departed, again and again, from the earlier authorities did he set them aside and rely on his own eyes. He dissected in the mortuaries, slaughter houses and hospitals, sometimes taking pieces back to his own rooms for further examination. He worked by day or by night, sometimes both – speed was essential – there were no refrigerators or baths of preservative, and it was a continuous race against the agents of putrefaction. To save time he kept a list of equipment he would need for a dissection, various itemised instruments, drawing materials and 'spectacles with the case'. He improved the lighting by making himself an oil lamp. Working in a pool of yellow light in the gloom of a mortuary with a malodorous corpse, Leonardo's dedication transcended what might well have been the repugnance felt by lesser mortals.

Leonardo was friendly with the monks at the hospital of Santa Maria Nuova, in Florence, who gave him access to the wards for both his artistic and anatomical work and provided him with facilities for dissection. Later, Pope Leo X (Giovanni de'Medici, the son of Lorenzo the Magnificent), allowed him to dissect at the hospital of Santo Spirito, in Rome, but after being accused of sacrilege by a rival for the Pope's patronage, the permission was withdrawn.

Leonardo made a thorough investigation of the human body, carrying out dissections on more than 30 bodies. He drew the bones and muscles, making sketches to show the mode of action of the body. He studied the nervous system, making meticulous drawings. His investigations of the alimentary canal, liver and blood system led him to puzzle over Galen's statement that blood was being made continuously in the liver. What happened to the blood? Surely the amount in the body at any one time must be constant? Was some of it being destroyed? He concluded that destroyed 'flesh' from organs returned in the blood vessels to the large intestine and contributed to the faeces. Leonardo was particularly interested in the heart and its mode of action, he made more drawings of it than any other organ. In one of his experiments on the heart, he tied off the attached blood vessels and injected air and then wax, in order to get an accurate idea of the shape and volume of the heart. Later, he made a glass model of the aorta and attached the valve ring and cusps from the aorta of an ox, fixing that in turn to a bag containing water to represent the ventricle. In the water were small grass seeds. On squeezing the bag he could simulate the flow of blood into the aorta, and the grass seeds showed the movement of currents passing the valve cusps. What he saw indicated that the aortic valve cusps close by pressure of eddying currents from the side, not by pressure brought about any tendency of the blood to be sucked back at the beginning of the phase of expansion (diastole). Whereas Galen had thought that diastole was the active movement of the heart, it is clear that Leonardo knew that it was contraction (systole), corresponding with the thump on the chest wall and causing the pulse. Nevertheless he thought that the force produced had spent itself by the time that the blood had reached the smaller vessels, so that he never discovered the circulation. Leonardo also noted the atria that Galen had mistaken for expanded regions at the origin of blood vessels, and ascribed the correct function to them: that of forcing the blood into the ventricles. It seemed to him, too, that as atria and ventricles were capable of contraction and relaxation, they must be composed of muscle; a fact which Galen had denied. Leonardo investigated Galen's theory that air entered the left ventricle from the lungs. He inflated the lungs hard and found that no air passed to the heart. All this left Galen's theories about the heart somewhat in disarray. Leonardo, however, believed, with Aristotle, that the heart was the source of heat distributed to the body. He reasoned in the following way: the atria contract forcing blood into the ventricles, these in turn contract driving blood into the pulmonary artery and aorta, but some is forced back into the atria. The movement of blood to and fro between the atria and ventricles creates friction, warming the blood. The warmed blood, in his view, rose to the head where it cooled and flowed back to the heart.

As Leonardo neared the end of his lifespan, the Spaniard, Miguel Serveto, or Servetus (1511–53), stood at the beginning of his. His father intended him to study law, but Servetus thought this too narrow a field. He had many interests: geography, theology, astronomy, mathematics and natural history, and he settled to study medicine instead, entering the University of Paris in 1536. This was the time of the rise of Protestantism, and Europe was going through a turbulent period. Servetus, a man of high intelligence and independence of mind, coupled with a passionate sincerity in his beliefs, was not far-seeing when it came to predicting the effect his radical views would have on his contemporaries. He made enemies of both Protestants and Catholics and fell out with the physicians in Paris. Eventually, he settled in a medical practice in Vienne, in south-west France. While he was studying medicine in Paris, he met the Protestant reformer, John Calvin, and continued to correspond with him, expressing open criticism of some aspects of bible teaching and making clear his rejection of the doctrine of the Trinity. Calvin, who broke off the correspondence, already had Servetus labelled, in his own mind, as a dangerous man.

During his medical studies, Servetus became convinced that pores in the interventricular septum of the heart, postulated by Galen, did not exist. He reached valid conclusions about the pulmonary circulation of the blood: in essence, he stated that blood is pumped out of the right ventricle to the lungs and then passes via anastomoses (proposed by Galen) to the veins and thence to the left ventricle and from there to all the arteries of the body. How did he reach these conclusions? Considering his intense interest in theological questions, it has been suggested that he accepted the literal truth of the statement in Genesis that God breathed his spirit into the heart of Adam, and with this in mind Servetus sought the site of the formation of the 'vital spirit', or 'breath of life', in man. Blood, suggested Servetus, met air in the lungs and changed from a dark red to a bright red before returning along the pulmonary veins to the left ventricle of the heart where it became 'vital spirit'. To Servetus, arterial blood was the 'vital spirit'.

In 1553, Servetus published his critical comments on the Bible, and his theories about the blood, in the volume *De Christianismi Restitutione* (On the Re-establishment of Christianity). He was foolish enough to send a copy to John Calvin. Calvin had already had dozens of people executed or thrown into prison for daring to dissent from his narrow and rigid views, and had decided that if ever Servetus visited Geneva, then under his control, he would not leave the town alive. He now acted swiftly and denounced Servetus to the Catholic Inquisition, making available Servetus's publication together with the private correspondence that had passed between them. Servetus was arrested, but taking advantage of incompetent guards, he managed to escape and hid in a monastery. After three months, he decided to make for Italy. One cannot imagine why he chose to travel through Geneva, but he did, and was recognised. Calvin showed him no mercy, keeping him in prison under unspeakable conditions for several months before bringing him to trial. He was allowed no one to defend him. 'A liar needs no defence', Calvin told him. Servetus was condemned to be burned at the stake and the fanatical Calvin ordered damp straw to be used to prolong his suffering. His books were burned with him; only four copies survive.

It was not until 1924 that an Egyptian doctor made the discovery that Ibn al-Nafis had described the pulmonary circulation of the blood, correctly, in the 13th century. It was considered to be unlikely that Servetus, who had been credited with the discovery in 1553, could possibly have known of his work. But a surprise was in store. Six years later, a Latin translation of some of the writings of Ibn al-Nafis were found. They had been published in Venice in 1547, and consisted of part of Ibn al-Nafis's *Commentary upon the Canon*, translated by Andrea Alpago, who made his own comments upon Galen's teaching about the heart and blood system together with Ibn al-Nafis's criticisms of it. The correlation of dates may be significant; on the other hand, Servetus may have come to his conclusions independently. It is interesting to note in passing that the Turkish science historian, Fuat Sezgin of Frankfurt University, currently engaged on a 20 volume work on the history of Arab science, provides ample evidence that in medieval times scientists in the West frequently pirated the work of Muslim scientists.

One of Servetus's fellow students at the University of Paris was Andreas van Wesele, or Vesalius (1514–64). He was born in Brussels, his father being court apothecary to the German Emperor, Charles V. As a child, Vesalius, who came of a family with a strong medical tradition, was eager to know how the human body worked, but for the time being he had to be content with animals. No animal was safe when Vesalius, with his overwhelming desire to explore its internal anatomy, set eyes upon it. Mice, rats, moles and squirrels revealed their secrets to his keen eye as he gained skill in dissection. Public executions were not uncommon in Vesalius's day and as he grew older he sought a good vantage point from which to view the proceedings, eagerly noting any details of scientific interest.

Vesalius began his studies at Louvain, finding no difficulty in learning Latin, Greek, Hebrew, Arabic and mathematics. He found Louvain rather conservative in outlook and moved on to Paris for his medical training. To his great disappointment he found Paris equally conservative, steeped in the Galenic tradition and with no opportunity for dissection. He worked hard and learned his work thoroughly, but he was eager to dissect and became impatient with his teachers. At this time France was at war with Germany, and soon there were enemy troops approaching Paris, so Vesalius, who had quarrelled with his teachers, took the opportunity to return to Louvain. It is said that during his stay in Paris he obtained corpses for dissection by all kinds of unorthodox means, and discovered anatomical details that did not correspond with those taught by Galen. On returning to Louvain he seems to have had some influence in the re-introduction of the practice of dissection that had been abandoned many years earlier. Vesalius obtained his medical qualifications in 1537, and at about this time he published a work on Rhazes. In the autumn of the same year he set off for Padua, in Italy.

The University of Padua was originally attached to the University of Bologna, established in 1113. The reputation of Padua had grown steadily and being close, geographically, to the Republic of Venice, it became officially associated with it. As the Republic of Venice was powerful, the University of Padua enjoyed a degree of freedom that helped it to become Italy's leading university. Students from a number of countries were attracted by its liberal policies and separate colleges were set up for the different nationalities.

On his way to Padua, Vesalius stopped in Venice. Here he met a fellow countryman, Jan Stephen van Calcar, a pupil of the artist, Titian, and together they journeyed to Padua. After taking examinations, Vesalius was granted the degree of Doctor of Medicine and was appointed to lecture on anatomy and surgery. He threw himself into the work with enthusiasm, performing the dissections personally as Mondino had done over two centuries before. To assist his students, Vesalius produced four large anatomical charts of the blood and nervous systems, annotated in Greek, Latin, Arabic and Hebrew. Later, having found that his chart of the nervous system had been copied and published, Vesalius published the other three together with three views of the skeleton. The drawings were by Jan Stephen van Calcar and the *Tabulae anatomicae sex*, was published in Venice in 1538. In the same year he published a dissection guide for the use of his students, and also visited Matthaeus Curtius, Professor of Medicine at Bologna, to discuss the practice of blood-letting or venesection.

At Padua, Vesalius was becoming a popular figure. Students flocked to his lectures and demonstration dissections. The bodies of criminals became available to him for dissection, and the more he dissected the clearer it became to him that there were an increasing number of anatomical points on which his observations differed from Galen. He came to realise that the differences were due to the fact that Galen had dissected the bodies of animals and then applied his findings to the human body. Vesalius, who hitherto had been moderately pro-Galen, now began to question Galen's views. The students of Bologna invited Vesalius to give them some anatomical demonstrations and he took the opportunity to emphasise that human anatomy could only be learned by observation and dissection of the human body. However, he also thought it wise not to neglect animal dissection, for it was helpful to observe the differences. Thus, he laid the foundations for the study of comparative anatomy.

On returning to Padua, Vesalius put all his time, energy and money into the preparation of a seven volume work on anatomy, employing the best possible draughtsmen and block cutters and supervising the production personally. The work, *De Humani Corporis Fabrica* (On the Structure of the Human Body), was printed by Joannes Oporinus of Basle and published in 1543. Vesalius firmly believed that a new approach was needed to the study of anatomy. 'There is little offered', he said, 'that could not better be taught by a butcher in his shop'. Had Vesalius only known of it, Leonardo's work on human anatomy was gathering dust in the home of Francesco Melzi, in Vaprio, near Milan. Vesalius's *De Fabrica* was greatly superior to earlier works. In it Vesalius had relied solely on his own observations, discarding misleading statements handed down from former authorities. It opened a new era in the study of anatomy and laid important foundations for modern medical science.

If Vesalius had expected acclaim, he was doomed to disappointment. In disgust he left Padua and applied to the Emperor Charles V, who appointed him physician to the Imperial household. Vesalius found the Emperor a difficult patient, but life had its compensations. In 1546, he married Anna van Hamme, daughter of a Brussels councillor, and he found it possible to keep up his research while travelling with the Emperor on his campaigns. He seized every opportunity to visit any medical schools nearby, he carried out post mortems, and he became a skilled military surgeon. His reputation spread and he came to be regarded as one of the great physicians of his time. After Charles V abdicated, Vesalius served with his son, Philip 11 of Spain, as physician to the Netherlanders at the Spanish court. Undoubtedly, the Inquisition had an eye on Vesalius and in 1564 he set out on a pilgrimage to Jerusalem. Tradition has it that only his royal patronage prevented more drastic measures being taken against him. However, on the return journey his ship was wrecked off the Greek island of Zakynthos and Vesalius lost his life.

In Book 3 of his *De Fabrica*, Vesalius's studies of the vascular system show he had encountered some difficulties probably owing to the rapidly putrefying material. In Book 5, dealing with the abdominal organs, he accepts Galen's view that blood is made in the liver. In Book 6, a work on the organs of the thorax, Vesalius suspects that the heart is composed of muscle, but says it cannot be true because its movement is involuntary. He regards the heart as a two-chambered structure, believing with his contemporaries that the atria were merely the bases of blood vessels. The presence of Galen's interventricular pores he thought very doubtful. In this volume he refers to the opinions of ancient philosophers regarding the soul, but refrains from comments of his own in case he should be regarded as 'suspect in his faith'. Is there any significance in the fact that Vesalius includes such considerations in his book concerning the heart? Had he the views of Aristotle in mind?

Successive occupants of the Chair of Anatomy and Surgery at Padua after Vesalius resigned, were Columbus, Fallopius and Fabricius. Each, in turn, corrected errors made by Vesalius, and published books of their own, all based on *De Fabrica*. Vesalius's insistence on the value of personal observation gradually diffused through Italy and from there throughout western Europe. His books were highly successful, and they, and illustrations from them, were widely plagiarised.

Vesalius had a high opinion of his assistant, Realdus Columbus (1516–80), who succeeded him at Padua. In 1559, Columbus published his work, *De re anatomica* (On Anatomy). He noted that the pulse in the arteries was exactly in time with the cardiac systole and demonstrated that the pulmonary veins contained bright red blood, not air. He gave his opinion that those believing in pores between the ventricles 'make a great mistake'. He repeated an experiment on an animal that Vesalius had performed; he noticed that with the lungs collapsed the heart beat was slow and sluggish, reviving when the lungs were reflated. Air, therefore, was very important. He was confident that blood passed by the pulmonary artery to the lungs and was returned with air by the pulmonary veins to the left ventricle of the heart. Clearly Columbus is describing the pulmonary circulation although, like his contemporaries, he did not recognise the atria as chambers of the heart. The question arises – was his belief in pulmonary circulation the result of his own original idea? In Columbus' favour is the fact that he had been taught by Vesalius, who attached great importance to personal observation, and Vesalius thought highly of him. Bearing this in mind, it seems improbable that Columbus would have been influenced by any physiological theories put forward in a theological work, published in 1553, by the impetuous radical Servetus, even if he knew of it, and that in itself is unlikely, as every effort was made to suppress his book. There remains the work of Ibn al-Nafis, published in Latin translation in Venice, in 1547. There is no evidence that Columbus knew of it although the dates could be regarded as uncomfortably close.

Columbus had a very able pupil by the name of Andreas Caesalpinus (1519–1603), who later published some important material. In 1571, Caesalpinus noted that the valves at the bases of the pulmonary artery and aorta allowed blood to flow in one direction only, and he deduced that blood passed from the right ventricle to the lungs, on to the left ventricle, and then to the aorta. In 1593, he published a further important discovery, observing that if a ligature were placed round the arm, blood collected in the veins on the distal side of the ligature, he concluded that the blood must be flowing towards the heart. He believed, with Galen, there must be anastomoses between the ends of the arteries and the ends of the veins, but appears to have had no conception of blood circulation. Although he actually uses the word 'circulation', it is quite clear that he failed to appreciate what caused the blood to move at all. In addition to his modern views, Caesalpinus held some that harked back to Aristotle. For example, he believed blood flowed along the arteries during the waking hours, but during sleep it carried heat back to the heart along the veins.

Gabriele Fallopius (1523–62), succeeded Columbus in the Chair of Anatomy and Surgery at Padua, in 1551. He is best known for his work on the inner ear and reproductive system. The tubes leading from the ovaries to the uterus, the Fallopian tubes, are named after him.

Succeeding Fallopius was Hieronymus Fabricius of Aquapendente (1537–1619). He had studied under Fallopius and obtained his diploma in 1559, giving private lessons in anatomy before being appointed to succeed Fallopius in 1565. Fabricius was a busy man; not only did he seek to improve methods of teaching his students, but he was much in demand as a skilled physician and surgeon as well as being a prolific writer on medical matters. Vesalius had demonstrated that it was often valuable to compare anatomical features in humans with the corresponding features in animals. Fabricius, who has been regarded as the Father of Comparative Anatomy, carried the idea much further and often spent demonstration time comparing structures in the human body with those in a number of different animals. His students, it seems, who were principally interested in passing their examinations, were impatient with what they regarded as unnecessary digressions and this led to noisy behaviour, earning irritated rebukes from Fabricius. If we assume that Plate V, showing Vesalius giving an anatomy demonstration, is typical of conditions at the time, we can imagine they were likely to have been an additional annoyance to Fabricius who set about designing a special theatre for anatomical demonstrations. The first was a wooden structure that could be erected and dismantled as required outside the building. In 1594, a permanent anatomy theatre, capable of holding over 200 students, was built. It consisted of five narrow circular galleries placed concentrically, each level being reached by means of a spiral staircase on the outside. Students stood in the galleries, leaning over a rail and looking down on the demonstration below – a marked improvement on the earlier system.

In 1609, a separate Chair of Surgery was created at Padua, and Fabricius remained as Professor of Anatomy until his retirement in 1613. Fabricius published a number of works on the plague, surgery, hearing, embryology, and one of particular interest to us, *De venarum ostiolis* (On the Valves in Veins). It was originally a separate publication of 1603, but was later incorporated with others under the general title *Opera anatomica* (Works on Anatomy), published in Padua in 1625. Fabricius tells us he first saw the valves in veins in 1574. He noticed they opened upwards and when filled with blood, would close and shut off a length of vein. He had no idea of their correct function, believing they served to slow down the flow of blood to the hands and feet.

Into the anatomy theatre at Padua, in January 1600, came a new student from England. He proved to be both talented and popular with his fellow students. In time he was to become more famous than his professor. His name was William Harvey.

Chapter 6

William Harvey (1578–1657)

At the time of William Harvey's birth in Folkestone, Kent, in 1578, a new era was beginning; Elizabeth 1 was establishing England as a Protestant kingdom, Francis Drake was sailing round the world and was destined to defeat the Spanish Armada, Francis Bacon, philosopher, scientist and future Lord Chancellor, was 17 years of age, and William Shakespeare had yet to make his name.

John Harvey, William's grandfather, was a prosperous sheep farmer who had set up Thomas, his son, with a farm of his own. Thomas made good, and in addition to his sheep farming he started a postal service in his area, later extending it to serve London and the French and Dutch coasts. In 1575, he married Joan Halke and three years later William was born. In due time William was to have six brothers and two sisters. Thomas had considerable business talent; he became associated with the Merchant Adventurers, trading not only in the Channel but as far away as the Levant. Four of William's brothers became wealthy merchants trading with Turkey, and another was associated with the court and became a Member of Parliament. William, it appears, came from a family who had brains and who knew how to use them. Did Thomas Harvey shrewdly observe that William's talents lay in directions other than business, or was it because he was the eldest son that he was placed in a position to climb the academic ladder? Or were there other reasons?

After attending a small local school, William Harvey

passed the examination for entry to the King's School, Canterbury, in 1588. At that time considerable emphasis was placed on Latin and Greek – scholars were expected to use no other language at work or at play. Harvey was undeterred by it and developed a deep appreciation of the great Latin poets. In 1569, Matthew Parker, Archbishop of Canterbury, provided sufficient funds for five scholarships to be awarded to scholars of the King's School; one was in medicine, tenable at Gonville and Caius College, Cambridge. It was one of the first scholarships in medicine ever to be awarded. Harvey won it at the age of 15.

Dr. John Caius (1510–73), had been a student at what was then Gonville Hall before leaving to study medicine at the University of Padua, Italy. During his stay in Padua, he became acquainted with Vesalius and by the time he returned to England he had become convinced of the importance of the study of anatomy. He was an enlightened man who also strove to improve the training of the barber-surgeons. His concern set in motion the process that was eventually to change the poor image of the Guild of Barber-Surgeons into a respected body of professional surgeons. He gave generously of his time and money to his old college which became Gonville and Caius. Dr. Caius and Archbishop Parker were friends and no doubt Dr. Caius was responsible for encouraging the Archbishop to endow a scholarship in medicine.

Harvey spent the first three years of his six-year scholarship period studying subjects that appear to bear little relationship to medicine. Thus, in 1597, he passed his Bachelor of Arts examination after studying theology, music, poetry, arithmetic, geometry and logic. Facilities for the study of medicine were apparently limited, for provision was made for study in Padua or other centres on the Continent. One needed to be physically tough to derive benefit from a university education in Harvey's time; there was no heating, the day began at 5 a.m. and continued until 9.30–10 p.m. with two short breaks for simple meals. In the second three-year period, Harvey appears to have been absent for long periods. In January 1600, he arrived at the University of Padua, his choice probably influenced by the fact that Dr. Caius had studied there. There is evidence that Harvey was well liked at both Cambridge and Padua. By its incorporation into the powerful Republic of Venice, Padua had gained greater freedom from control by the Church. It suited Harvey well, and he warmed to its intellectual freedom and its respect for the views of Aristotle and some of the Arabic physicians. He was already well versed in the work of Vesalius and came to be greatly influenced by the work of Vesalius' successors, Columbus, Fallopius, and his own professor, Fabricius d'Aquapendente.

Harvey graduated from Padua in 1602, and returned to London. Two years later he married Elizabeth Brown, daughter of a court physician. There were no children of the marriage. William and Elizabeth lived near St Paul's Cathedral, within a short distance of five of William's brothers, and also, after 1605, of his father who moved nearby after the death of his wife. The male members of the family appear to have remained close all their lives. In 1607, Harvey was elected a Fellow of the College of Physicians, and two years later he was appointed Physician to St. Bartholomew's Hospital. For over 30 years Harvey visited the hospital at least once a week, examining each patient and writing out a prescription for the apothecary to dispense. In 1613, Harvey was elected a Censor of the College of Physicians, giving him power to supervise physicians in London and to enter any apothecary's premises to inspect his apparatus and medicinal materials. Clearly, the College of Physicians thought highly of Harvey: in 1616 he was invited to give the Lumleian lectures, and he continued to do so until a year before his death; in 1627, the College made him an Elect, with responsibility for the examination of physicians wishing to practise medicine in London, while the following year saw him become Treasurer of the College.

Meanwhile, in 1618, Harvey had been appointed Physician Extraordinary to King James 1, and when Charles 1 succeeded his father to the throne in 1625, he retained Harvey in that post. Harvey became Physician in Ordinary five years later. King Charles became a close friend of Harvey's, taking a great personal interest in his work on animal anatomy and making sure he was supplied with deer for his observations. Harvey, in his turn, took pains to point out features of special interest to the King; their shared enthusiasm cemented a lasting friendship. Harvey made a number of journeys overseas on behalf of the King, a matter of some displeasure to the Governors of St. Bartholomew's Hospital. On one such occasion, in 1636, that took him near Venice, Harvey found himself falling foul of the Venetian quarantine regulations. Owing to some irregularity in his *fede di sanita*, a pass certifying that he was free of plague, he was confined in quarantine for two weeks. Harvey shows in his letters of complaint to Basil Fielding, King Charles's Ambassador Extraordinary to the Republic of Venice, that he was quite capable of being very angry indeed. Surprisingly, in spite of his understandable annoyance, nowhere do we find even a glimpse of recognition that such regulations were an enlightened measure for the time.

In 1639, Harvey was promoted to Senior Physician in Ordinary to the King, and was provided with rooms in Whitehall. Charles 1 was on the throne at a time when the ordinary people were beginning to feel their power. Parliament challenged the King's view of his own divine right, and for both political and religious reasons a great rift appeared between the King and his supporters on the one hand, and Parliament and the Puritans on the other. Harvey remained steadfastly Royalist, while he looked on sadly at the King's declining fortunes. Civil war erupted in 1642, and Harvey suffered a personal loss in the early days when a mob, looting houses belonging to Royalists, wrecked his own apartment in Whitehall. His furniture and books he could replace, but his notes covering observations over 40 years of professional life were irreplaceable, and their loss caused him great grief.

Harvey, having largely withdrawn from St. Bartholomew's Hospital, perhaps because of the unpopularity of his support for the Royalist cause, was with the King at the Battle of Edgehill, where, Aubrey has it, he sat under a hedge 'and tooke out of his pockett a booke and read'. (John Aubrey (1626–97), was a friend of Harvey's.) Charles 1 then made his headquarters at Oxford for the next four years, and Harvey was elected Warden of Merton College. The previous Warden had absented himself for some time and the Fellows of the College were disposed to elect a replacement. To the King, they presented their nominations which included the name of William Harvey. The King replied, 'Wee doe choose our Welbeloved Servant Dr. William Harvey, one of our principall physitians to be your Warden . . .'

A great change was to take place in Harvey life after the execution of Charles 1, in 1649. The King's death left a gap in his life and he turned his attention more and more to the affairs of the College of Physicians. He had built, at his own expense, a handsome new library and museum for the benefit of the College. In the same year he was elected President, but he declined the honour feeling that his health was not up to the strain. He died in 1657, in the home of his brother, Eliab, in Roehampton and was buried in the family vault in Hempstead, Essex.

During his lifetime, Harvey published two important works; *De Motu Cordis et Sanguinis in Animalbus* (Movement of the Heart and Blood in Animals), in which he put forward his theory of the circulation of the blood, and *De Generatione Animalium* (Animal Generation). It seems likely that Harvey came to his conclusions about the circulation of the blood over a period of time. His notes for the Lumleian lectures, the *Prelectiones*, are dated 1616, and it is possible that Harvey made a tentative suggestion about the blood circulation when making a demonstration dissection of the chest cavity in 1618. There are possible reasons why Harvey might not wish to reveal all he knew; on the other hand, the particular notes referring to circulation may have been added at a later date, as some historians believe. Why would Harvey wish to keep such an important discovery to himself? We have to use imagination and put ourselves back into the 17th century: at that time authority was all, and the authority of Galen still lay heavily on the study of medicine – to challenge Galen's views was to invite discredit and abuse. The whole mood of the time was different – public executions were commonplace and belief in witchcraft prevalent, even among physicians. Harvey himself had been commanded by Charles 1 to be present at the examination of several women accused of witchcraft. Furthermore, at the time Harvey commenced to give the Lumleian lectures, only 63 years had passed since Servetus had been burned at the stake for his views. The environment in Harvey's day was not entirely congenial for the scientist.

Dr. Kenneth Keele, in his book *William Harvey, the Man, the Physician and the Scientist*, describes Harvey as a 'reluctant revolutionary'. He believes that Harvey, educated in the classics, orthodox in ambition, conventional in behaviour and a loyal supporter of the Royal cause, would have found it difficult to publicise his revolutionary ideas about the circulation of the blood. His discovery would overthrow the authority of Galen, and he would be fully aware of the consequences. On the other hand, his integrity would demand that he make his discoveries known.

With the exception of the enlightened views of Vesalius that had penetrated anatomy teaching in Padua, Harvey's medical education had proceeded along orthodox lines; that is, they had been based on the works of Galen. Harvey, however, rejected Galen's physiology and turned to Aristotle. He was very much in harmony with the intellect of Aristotle, who had been one of the first to carry out animal dissections and record his detailed observations, and who had also laid great emphasis on the heart as the centre of physical and mental processes. Harvey was also influenced by his professor, Fabricius, who was himself a great supporter of Aristotle.

It seems that in clinical practice, Harvey's approach was conventional. Had it not been so, it is unlikely that he would have risen to high office in the College of Physicians. There is evidence that he was not against blood-letting, believing the practice had 'a most salutary effect in many diseases', and he condemned notions of possible blood transfusions as worthless. Most physicians in Harvey's day carried out a rather perfunctory examination of the patient, and Harvey appears to have been no exception. The now routine temperature check and pulse count were not features of a clinical examination, although the necessary instruments existed.

Nevertheless, in *De Motu Cordis,* Harvey reveals the mind of a modern scientist in his clear reasoning, careful observation, anatomical investigations and quantitative assessments. It is well worth following the reasoning behind his theory of the circulation of the blood, set out in his book. Harvey says that the movement of the heart can be observed in the exposed heart of a living mammal, but that it is difficult to distinguish between diastole and systole, these phases of the heart's action being more readily observable in cold-blooded animals such as amphibians, or in a mammal when the heart is slowing down and failing. He observed systole to be a contraction of the heart, noting that it became hard to the touch like tensed muscles in the forearm when the fingers are moved, also that at this time it became paler in colour. This convinced him, in spite of Galen's opposing view, that systole was the active phase of the heartbeat and the one that, by the upward movement of the heart, caused it to strike the chest wall, a movement that could be felt and heard. Harvey clearly regards the heart as muscle, contracting in systole and forcing blood into the arteries, causing them to expand and produce a pulse. He notes that if a ventricle wall is pierced or an artery cut during systole, blood spurts out. He observes that the atria contract together, followed by simultaneous contraction of the two ventricles. This was in opposition to the contemporary view, but had been observed by Leonardo da Vinci. Harvey reveals that he made observations on over 80 different species of animals, from invertebrates to mammals. (This is very much in the tradition of Aristotle.) He totally refuted Galen's theory of the interventricular pores saying: 'There are no pores and it is not possible to show such'. To Harvey, the heart is clearly a pump. Pumps for water were not uncommon in Harvey's time, and would have been known to him.

Turning to the distribution of blood in the body, Harvey notes that in the foetus, blood passes directly from the right ventricle to the left ventricle through an opening, the *foramen ovale,* which closes at birth. He also observes the *ductus arteriosus* joining the pulmonary and aortic arches, and serving to transfer blood from the right ventricle to the aorta.

In some animals, he records, these structures remain open for varying periods of time and sometimes for life. If blood passes from the right ventricle to the left ventricle in animals without lungs, and in the foetus, which has no functional lungs, what is the route when the lungs function and the *foramen ovale* and *ductus arteriosus* close? Harvey asked himself. He concluded it must be through the lungs. Furthermore, he argues that only one ventricle is necessary in animals without lungs, the second only becoming required when the blood has to pass through the lungs. (Harvey does not show that he appreciates why passage through the lungs should be necessary.)

Harvey's opponents were quick to point out that none of this proved that blood did not pass through interventricular pores, as Galen had stated. Later, Harvey set out to settle this point. Taking the corpse of a man, he ligatured the pulmonary artery, pulmonary veins and the aorta, and opened the left ventricle. He then forced a quantity of water through the vena cavae so that the right atrium and right ventricle were greatly distended. No water escaped from the opening he had made in the left ventricle. Next, he untied the ligatures from the pulmonary artery and veins, forced more water through the vena cavae, whereupon water and blood gushed from the opening in the left ventricle.

Harvey had gradually been coming to the conclusion that far too much blood was being pumped out by the heart to make Galen's view that it was continuously being produced in the liver, credible. 'I began privately to consider', he says, 'if it had a movement, as it were, in a circle'. He decided to estimate the quantity of blood passing through the heart in a given time. In modern terms, his calculations were along these lines: in a human about $60cm^3$ of blood are transmitted with each heart beat, this would amount to 250 litres an hour and would weigh over 200 kilogrammes, three times the weight of an average man. It was clear to him that the same blood must be circulating! The presence of one-way valves in the heart and blood vessels had already coaxed his mind along these channels. Valves are not present in veins, he says, to prevent blood collecting in the lower parts, as Fabricius had taught, but to guide the blood towards the centre of the body. The valves in the jugular vein in the neck, he noted, face downwards.

Using illustrations borrowed from Fabricius (Plate IX), Harvey says that if a ligature is tied round the upper arm and the blood is pressed out of a length of vein by drawing the finger along from O to H, one finger being held at H, no blood flows from O to fill the gap. If now a finger is pressed down above the valve at O, no blood can be forced through the valve. If the finger is now lifted from H, the empty portion of the vein is filled from the side away from the heart.

It is significant that Harvey's work was entitled *Movement of the Heart and Blood in Animals*. He could demonstrate the movement, but he could not demonstrate that blood circulated; it was a theory. The mystery of how blood flowed from the arteries back into the veins remained, and in spite of extensive research, Harvey could find no connections between them. That mystery remained to be solved, and by the time it was, Harvey was dead.

The reaction provoked by the publication of Harvey's *De Motu Cordis*, in 1628, was typical of that accorded to the works of one far in advance of his time. Harvey had anticipated the disbelief, abuse and criticism of his experiments, and the ignoring of his discoveries. Medical teaching continued to proceed along orthodox lines, and he received little support. Even in his own country his theory took more than 20 years to gain acceptance. However, he was luckier than some: he did live to see his theory accepted.

In 1651, Harvey published his *De Generatione Animalium*. In it he set out to clarify the reproduction of animals and to compare his findings with those of Aristotle, and of his professor at Padua, Fabricius. In it his scientific findings are interwoven with a large content of philosophical matter.

Chapter 7

Studies with the Microscope

Harvey's account of the circulation of the blood had to remain a theory, for, in spite of every effort, he had been unable to demonstrate how blood from the arteries got back into the veins. But even while Harvey was in his thirties, developments were taking place in Holland which were to lead to the last piece of the jigsaw falling into place.

One day in 1608, a young man apprenticed to the optician and lens grinder, Hans Lippershey (1587–1619), was toying with some of his master's lenses and while holding two in front of his eyes and moving them back and forth he found, to his surprise, that distant objects appeared closer. Lippershey at once saw the significance of his observation and setting to work with enthusiasm he mounted two suitable lenses in a tube, so making the first telescope. He tried to interest the Dutch government in the invention, but they were unimpressed. Within a year, news of the telescope had drifted through to Padua and reached the ears of Galileo (1564–1642). He was greatly excited by the news, and before many months had passed he had made himself a telescope with a magnification of 32. With his simple telescope he saw what had never been seen before: sunspots, satellites around the planet Jupiter and phases of Venus like those of the moon. He also found that by rearranging the lenses it was possible to view small objects close at hand, and he looked at insects seeing details of their structure not visible before. He had made a microscope! He sent one of his telescopes to the German astronomer, Johann Kepler (1571–

1630), who, by 1611, described both an improved telescope and an improved microscope. This type of microscope, with more than one lens, was the forerunner of the modern compound microscope, but the early ones with their imperfect lenses were limited in their definition and magnification, and improvement came slowly.

In the same year that Harvey published his *De Motu Cordis*, Marcello Malpighi (1628–94), was born in Crevalcore, near Bologna. He studied medicine and philosophy at the University of Bologna, graduating in 1653. At first he lectured in logic at Bologna, but in 1656, he was offered the chair in theoretical medicine at the University of Pisa. However, he did not like the climate, and after three years he returned to a similar post in Bologna. An offer of the chair of medicine at the University of Messina tempted him south for four years, and then his beloved Bologna drew him back again, until, at the age of 63, he reluctantly retired to Rome as physician to Pope Innocent XII. Malpighi was drawn to the new invention, the early compound microscope, and he began his studies in microscopy in the 1650s. Having the advantage of a medical training, he was well placed to carry out a planned programme of research and to evaluate the results. He soon showed himself to be a master of microscope technique and he is usually regarded as the Father of Microscopy. In 1667, the Royal Society in London invited him to communicate his research findings to them, and this he continued to do for many years. The Royal Society elected him a Fellow in 1668, and supervised the printing of his later works.

One of Malpighi's early investigations concerned the lungs. At that time they were regarded as rather fleshy structures, but Malpighi showed that they consisted of thin membranes covering vast numbers of minute air sacs, the membranes having a rich network of very fine blood vessels. He believed that minute arteries and air tubes opened into the air sacs and that a mixture of blood and air entered the openings of minute veins. He examined other parts of the body for connections between arteries and veins, before turning to frogs' lungs, which are more transparent. Here he was able to see that blood passed from arteries to veins in tiny hair-like tubes, and he found the same in the bladder. Blood capillaries were revealed for the first time! Here, before his eyes, was the answer to the problem that Harvey had sought for so long, the final piece of information which proved Harvey's theory. He published his findings in 1661. Four years later, in a publication dealing with membranes, Malpighi described red-coloured fat globules in the blood vessels (presumably these were red blood cells).

In his research into the anatomy of insects, Malpighi discovered the tracheae, the branching tubes that open to the outside in the abdomen and through which the insect obtains oxygen for respiration. In 1669, he published a book about silkworms, giving a full account of the spiracles, tracheae, nerve cord, silk glands and reproductive system. Two works on the chick embryo followed, *De formatione pulli in ova* (On the formation of the chick in the egg), in 1672 and *De ovo incubato* (On the incubated egg), in 1675. Whatever the reasons may have been, it is clear that he did not see the earliest stages of development, and therefore he came to the conclusion that the parts of the chick were present from the beginning, and merely enlarged and unfolded. This 'pre-formation' theory was a red herring which drew a number of scientists off the trail, and even resulted in a little preformed man being 'seen' (and drawn) in a human sperm cell, and tiny embryos being 'found' in mammalian ova. Turning from animals to plants, Malpighi published two volumes on plant anatomy in 1675 and 1679, which were classics of that era. Further research into the organs and structures of the human body followed, and Malpighi became very skilled in his preparation of material for the microscope, examining muscle, bone, brain, kidney and liver tissue, the spinal cord, nerves and skin. His name is still associated with the dividing layer in the skin (Malpighian layer) and the blind end of the uriniferous tubule with its bunch of capillaries (Malpighian body) in the kidney. Malpighi was a pioneer in the field of scientific microscopy. He studied such a wide range of material that the curiosity of many workers with varying interests was aroused and many valuable discoveries were made.

Meanwhile, in Holland, the home of Hans Lippershey, surprising events were taking shape. On the face of it, one would hardly expect a cloth merchant to make the totally independent discovery of the 'anastomoses' between arteries and veins that Harvey had striven so hard to find, but Anton van Leeuwenhoek (1632–1723), was no ordinary cloth merchant. He was born in Delft and apprenticed to a linen merchant in Amsterdam. Five years later, when he was 21, he returned to his home town, set up on his own as a draper and got married. He augmented his income by service, in a part-time capacity, at the local town hall. Leeuwenhoek, however, was not content solely with this conventional existence, he had an obsessive hobby – lens grinding. Opticians had a good reputation in Holland and Leeuwenhoek learned the craft from them. He worked at his grinding bench, shaping and polishing to perfection each tiny biconvex lens, some scarcely more than pinhead sized. Taking a lens, he secured it between small holes in two rectangular metal plates, and delighted in its magnification. The object to be examined he mounted on a silver needle connected to a screw mechanism to bring it to the correct focus. Holding his own carefully made microscope close to his eye, he marvelled at everything he saw: exquisite scales from a butterfly's wing, sculptured pollen grains, tiny insects and the assortment of fibres and particles making up a speck of dust. He used capillary tubes to hold liquid for examination; drops of pond water revealed a complete new world of plants and animals far too small to be seen with the unaided eye. Leeuwenhoek was enthralled. He improved the illumination by adding a small concave mirror and he was the first person ever to see bacteria – he found them first in water and in tooth scrapings.

In 1673, Leeuwenhoek wrote to the Royal Society in London, to report his findings. This august body was accustomed to dealing with learned gentlemen at home and overseas, but they must have received his communication with some incredulity. However, Leeuwenhoek also sent some of his microscopes so that the scholarly Fellows might see for themselves. Robert Hooke (1635–1703), an eminent physicist and biologist who was Secretary of the Royal Society at the time, made some microscopes to Leeuwenhoek's specification. For the next 50 years, Leeuwenhoek corresponded with the Royal Society reporting his discoveries and observations about all manner of things: protozoa, rotifers, volvox, yeast, and the life histories of various insects and marine and freshwater mussels. One hundred and fifty extracts from his letters were published in the *Philosophical Transactions* between 1673 and 1723. By a unanimous vote he was elected a Fellow of the Royal Society in 1680.

One day, Leeuwenhoek examined the delicate tail of a live tadpole through his lenses noticing very fine blood vessels that formed a connection between artery and vein, and he described how each vessel possessed a turning point where the blood completed its outward journey and began to return to the heart. He also noticed that blood was not a homogeneous fluid but contained lots of identical rounded bodies. He described his findings to the Royal Society in even more precise detail than Malpighi had done.

When Leeuwenhoek died, he left nearly 250 microscopes and about 200 lenses. To the Royal Society he bequeathed a cabinet with 26 microscopes together with extra lenses which had a magnification of 50–250. These microscopes have since disappeared from the Royal Society's collection. Considering the detailed accounts and drawings of the 'smallest animalcules' that Leeuwenhoek sent to the Royal Society, it is likely that some of the lenses he used had a greater magnification. Whatever his secrets, the tough little Dutchman, lacking in formal education, butt of his neighbours' jests, was privileged to see into a new world, observing, marvelling and meticulously recording all he saw. His achievements caught the public imagination, Peter the Great of Russia and Queen Mary of England visited him, and he became world famous.

When Malpighi reported his findings of red-coloured fat globules in blood vessels, he would have been unaware that Jan Swammerdam (1637–80), a Dutch naturalist, had already observed the same phenomenon. Swammerdam looked at the blood of different kinds of animals and noticed that all the reddish blobs were of the same size and shape. When he examined frogs' blood he found that all the blobs had a structure in the centre (red blood cells in the frog are nucleated). He realised that these reddish blobs were an integral part of the blood, and that it was not a homogeneous liquid as others had supposed. He reported his observations in 1658, when he was only 21.

Jan Swammerdam was born in Amsterdam, the son of an apothecary who collected natural curiosities. As a boy, Jan helped his father collect specimens and arrange them in his museum, and this gave him a lifelong interest in natural history, with a particular passion for insects. He studied medicine at the University of Leyden, graduating in 1667, but it is doubtful if he ever practised, in spite of pressure from his father. Instead, he collected over 3,000 specimens of insects, and was lost in wonder at their beauty and variety, and the exquisite perfection of their tiny bodies. He made a study of the micro-anatomy of many different species, producing excellent drawings, not superseded today. He published a general history of insects in 1669, and an account of the structure of the mayfly in 1675. Unfortunately for science, in 1673, he came under the influence of a Flemish religious fanatic, Antoinette Bourignon, and became increasingly drawn away from his microscopy into the religious controversy associated with her cult. Nevertheless, even in his short academic life, his work earned him the title of Father of Entomology. Fortunately, 50 years after his death, his manuscripts and drawings were purchased by Hermann Boerhaave, a Dutch physician who published them, at his own expense, in two volumes, *Biblia naturae* (Bible of Nature), in 1737. In these volumes, the text of which was translated into Latin, Swammerdam provides the first scientific account of insect metamorphosis. For each selected insect he gives an account of the life history and details of the anatomy. He was the first to describe accurately the mouthparts, compound eyes and sting of the honey bee.

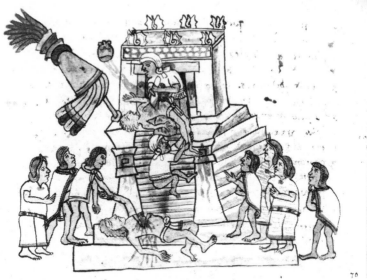

I Sacrifice to the Sun God. An Aztec warrior is held down while a priest cuts out his heart. An earlier victim is seen at the foot of the steps. (BIBLIOTECA NAZIONALE CENTRALE, FLORENCE.)

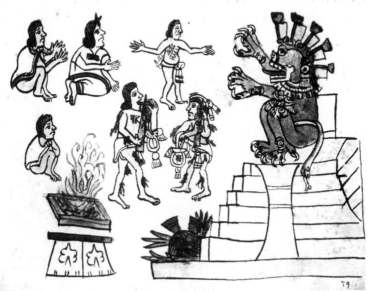

II Aztec worshippers offer blood from self-inflicted wounds to the God of the Dead. (BIBLIOTECA NAZIONALE CENTRALE, FLORENCE.)

III
Right: *Galen (130–200 AD).*
From a work by Ambroise
Paré. (ROYAL COLLEGE OF
PHYSICIANS, LONDON.)

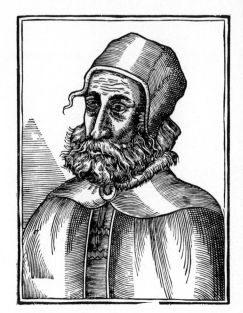

IV
Below: *Drawings of the heart*
of an ox, by Leonardo da Vinci
(1452–1519). (ROYAL
LIBRARY, WINDSOR CASTLE.)

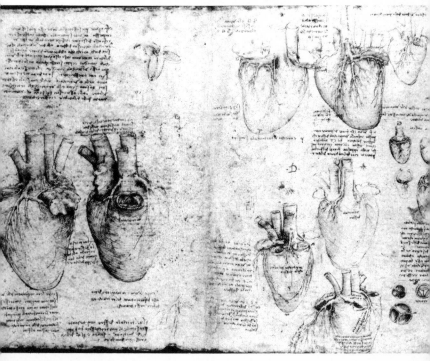

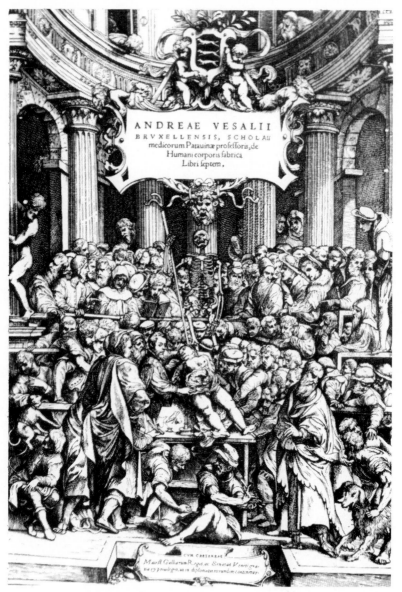

V Title page of the first edition of Vesalius's De Humani Corporis Fabrica
*(Basle 1543). (*WAYLAND PUBLISHERS LTD.*)*

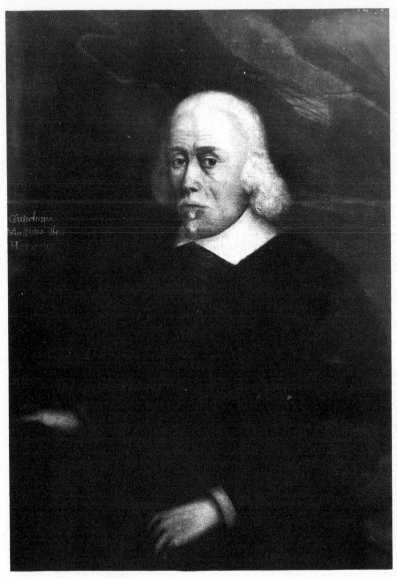

VI William Harvey (1578–1657), from a portrait in possession of the National Portrait Gallery, London. (MANSELL COLLECTION.)

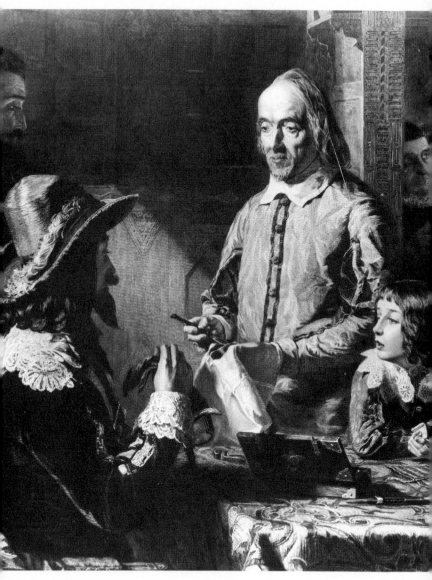

VII 'Harvey demonstrates to Charles 1 his theory of the circulation of the blood'. From a painting by Robert Hannah. (MANSELL COLLECTION.)

EXERCITATIO
ANATOMICA DE
MOTV CORDIS ET SAN-
GVINIS IN ANIMALI-
BVS,

GVILIELMI HARVEI ANGLI,
Medici Regii, & Professoris Anatomiæ in Col-
legio Medicorum Londinensi.

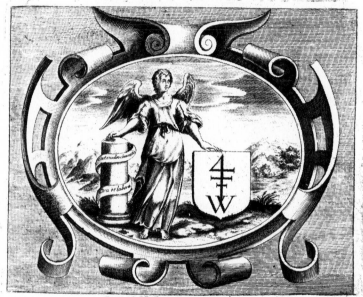

FRANCOFVRTI,
Sumptibus GVILIELMI FITZERI.

ANNO M. DC. XXVIII.

VIII *Title page of William Harvey's* De Motu Cordis et Sanguinis in
Animalibus *(Frankfurt 1628).* (THE BRITISH LIBRARY.)

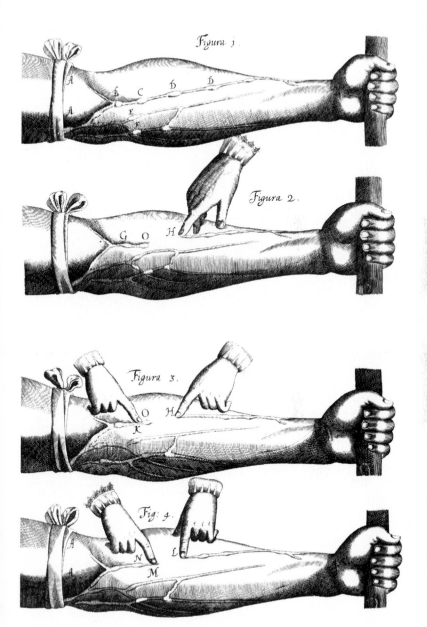

IX Illustrations from William Harvey's De Motu Cordis *demonstrating the circulation of the blood.* (THE BRITISH LIBRARY.)

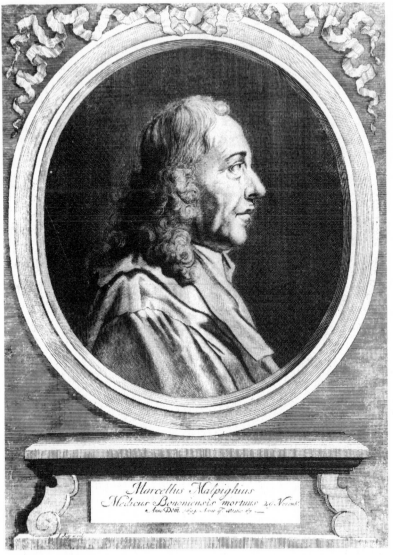

Marcellus Malpighius

Medicus Bononiensis mortuus 26 Novemb.
Anno Dom. 1694. Anno ætatis 66.

X *Marcello Malpighi (1628–94), from his* Opera Omnia. (ROYAL COLLEGE
OF PHYSICIANS, LONDON.)

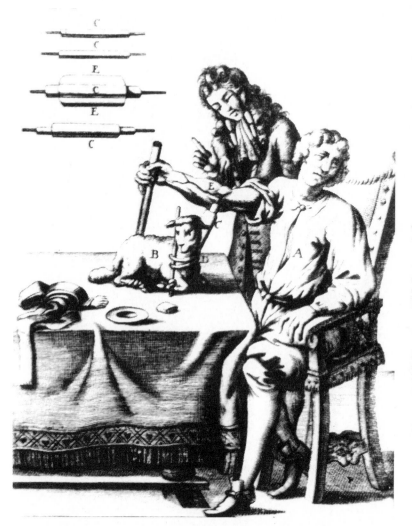

XI *A blood transfusion from animal to human. An illustration from* Gierbluttransfusion *by M. G. Purmann (1648–1721).* (BILDARCHIV PREUSSISCHER KULTURBESITZ, BERLIN.)

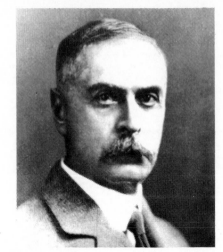

XII **Right:** *Karl Landsteiner (1868–1943).* (WELLCOME INSTITUTE.)

XIII **Below:** *X-ray diffraction pattern of horse haemoglobin.* (DR. MAX PERUTZ.)

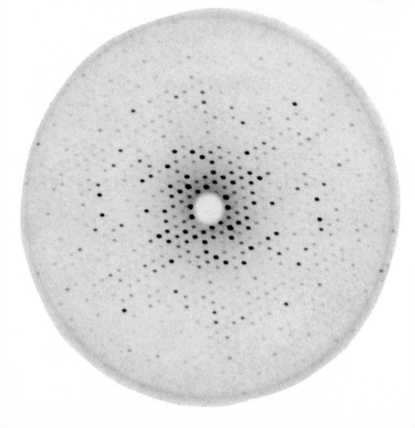

Chapter 8

The Advance of Experimental Physiology

Once Harvey's theory of the circulation of the blood had been accepted, one might have expected spectacular advances to be made in medicine, but this was not the case. The reason lay in the fact that physics and chemistry had not advanced far enough for their findings to be applied to living systems. As far as practical applications were concerned, after one or two abortive attempts to make use of it, Harvey's theory lay in cold storage. Some physicians saw the possibility of injecting medicines of various kinds directly into the veins, and discussions took place within the Royal Society on this matter. The possibility of transfusing blood from one animal to another, an idea suggested by Sir Christopher Wren, was also discussed. Wren's fame as the architect of the new St. Paul's Cathedral and other famous churches, has obscured the fact that he was a leading scientist of the day, and was at one time President of the Royal Society.

Richard Lower (1631–91), had already experimented with the injection of liquids into the veins of animals, and in 1666, he demonstrated the direct transfusion of blood from an artery of one dog into a vein of another. His experiment, the first successful blood transfusion, was reported in the *Philosophical Transactions*. Richard Lower was born in Cornwall and studied medicine at Oxford, where he proved very adept at dissection, often preparing dissections for his professor, Thomas Willis, who thought highly of him. After obtaining his medical qualifications, Lower moved to

London and built up a successful practice. His experiments in blood transfusion led to his election as a Fellow of the Royal Society. Jean Denys (1625–1704), a professor at the University of Montpellier, read of Lower's experiments and, in 1667, he succeeded in transfusing the blood of a lamb into a patient. Encouraged by this first success, he followed it with several others. Later on, in the same year, Lower performed a similar experiment, the first successful blood transfusion from animal to man, in England. The jubilation was short lived, however, for one of Denys's patients died, and as legal proceedings followed, blood transfusion experiments were abandoned for well over a century. Another experiment Lower performed was to inject venous blood into an inflated lung and observe that the previously dark colour of the blood changed to a bright red. From this, he drew the conclusion that the colour change was due to the mixing of the blood with air. He suspected that something from the air was absorbed by the blood, but ideas about what that might be had to wait another century.

Up to the second half of the 17th century there had been few quantitative experiments on the heart and blood system. Harvey's was a notable exception, for he had shown by means of two basic measurements on man, that blood must be circulating round the body. He had counted the number of heart beats in a given time, and he had also recorded the volume of blood found in the left ventricle of a cadaver: as we have seen, a simple calculation revealed that in one hour, the weight of blood pumped out by the heart was three times that of the weight of the man, and that was clearly impossible unless the blood was circulating. Like most brilliant ideas, it appears deceptively simple in hindsight.

Another Englishman, the Reverend Stephen Hales (1677–1761), took a major step forward in the physiological field. Science was his hobby and he was a great admirer of Sir Isaac Newton, whose precise measurements and calculations had convinced Hales that the way forward in biology was to use quantitative methods to solve problems. Many of Hales' experiments were conducted with plants; he is considered to be the founder of plant physiology. He possessed an inventive mind; among his ideas was a method of obtaining fresh water from sea water, and a way of keeping grain free of insect attack by the use of sulphur dioxide. In 1727, he published a book about his discoveries which was sufficiently well thought of to secure his election to the Royal Society. In 1733, Hales made the first successful measurement of blood pressure. He determined the pressure in the main artery and main vein in the neck of a horse. On inserting a long glass tube into the carotid artery he found that the blood rose in the tube to a height of 2.92 metres, whereas inserted into the jugular vein, the blood rose to a height of only 0.5 metres. To Hales, this showed the importance of the pressure in the aorta in driving the blood round the body. He then set about finding out just how much blood flowed from the heart of the horse in one minute. He noted the number of heart beats per minute, and that was 36. Next, he bled the horse to death (animal experiments in those days were not covered by the strict regulations that are in force today), and determined the capacity of the left ventricle by pouring melted wax into it and allowing it to solidify. On removal, he found its volume to be 160 cm^3. A simple calculation for the blood flow, 36 x 160, gave him the figure of 5.8 litres per minute. In fact, although the method he used was sound the result was inaccurate – the heart muscle had contracted strongly on death, thus considerably reducing the capacity of the ventricle.

The 18th century was the time of the phlogiston theory. It was believed that combustible matter contained phlogiston which was lost on burning, leaving an incombustible residue; air merely served as a means of carrying away the phlogiston or transferring it to something else. It was thought that the rusting of iron was a form of combustion, but problems arose when it was discovered that rusting iron gained weight, whereas when most materials burned they lost it! In 1775, Joseph Priestley (1733–1804), an English chemist with a keen interest in gases, took some of the red calx (mercuric oxide) that formed on heating mercury, and heated it separately. He was surprised to find that shining globules of mercury reappeared, and at the same time a gas was given off that caused burning materials to burn more brightly. Priestley had discovered oxygen, but he, believing in the phlogiston theory of the time, called it 'dephlogisticated air'. Karl Scheele (1742–86), a Swedish chemist, had also discovered oxygen independently, a few years before, but owing to tardiness on the part of his publisher it did not appear in print until 1777.

It took the clear-sighted French chemist, Antoine-Laurent Lavoisier (1743–94), to debunk the phlogiston theory and to make discoveries of profound importance to biology. Lavoisier believed that materials burned well in Priestley's 'dephlogisticated air' for the simple reason that it was not mixed with the part of the air that did not support combustion. He had already carried out some experiments with mercury calx and now he extended the work. First, he heated mercury in air in such a way that no fresh supply of air could reach it. He continued the heating for a long time and then examined the residual air. Would it allow a candle to burn in it? No, so something had been lost from the air. Did it give a precipitate with lime water? No, therefore it was not carbon dioxide. He then mixed five parts of the residual air with one part of Priestley's 'dephlogisticated air' and found that a candle burned in it with the same degree of brightness as in ordinary air. By 1778, he was confident enough to state that air consisted of two gases, one in which substances would burn, he named it 'oxygen', and one in which they would not.

Lavoisier found that birds lived quite happily in oxygen, but at the same time they released carbon dioxide into it. He demonstrated that carbon would burn in oxygen to produce carbon dioxide, and he also repeated an experiment first performed by Henry Cavendish (1731–1810), an English chemist and physicist, who showed that water was formed when hydrogen was burned in air. By now, suspicions were forming in Lavoisier's mind that breathing most likely led to a process similar to combustion. Soon, he voiced his belief that in breathing, only oxygen was involved, the rest of the air entering and leaving the lungs unchanged. One of two things happened when animals breathed, he believed, either the oxygen was converted to carbon dioxide in the lungs, or the oxygen was absorbed and an approximately equal volume of carbon dioxide supplied by the lungs. He favoured the first alternative as being similar to combustion. This, he argued, was accompanied by the release of heat and would account for the production of animal heat. In 1790–91, Lavoisier and Seguin showed that in an animal the quantity of oxygen consumed increased with temperature, and during digestion and exercise.

Lavoisier divided his time between his scientific research and his duties as a public servant. In addition to being a brilliant chemist and an able financier, he was actively interested in geology, advocated a more scientific approach to agriculture, and was a humanitarian who served on a number of boards and committees formed to help the poor and unfortunate. But none of it was to save him from a terrible end. During the French Revolution, Jean-Paul Marat, a revolutionary leader who harboured a grudge against Lavoisier, had him arrested on trifling and absurd charges, and his reputation failed to save him from the guillotine. Lagrange, a celebrated Italian-French astronomer and mathematician, said sorrowfully, 'It took them only an instant to cut off that head and a hundred years may not produce another like it'. Only two years later, the remorseful French were honouring the memory of one of the greatest martyrs of the time.

Lavoisier's brilliantly planned series of experiments showed that an animal takes oxygen from the surrounding air for a vital process, a combustion, within its living body, producing heat and waste carbon dioxide. He was mistaken only in believing that combustion took place in the lungs. This was corrected by Claude Bernard (1813–78), a French physiologist and pioneer of experimental physiology. After he left school, Bernard became apprenticed to an apothecary, but after the initial enthusiasm had worn off he found himself thoroughly bored with the daily routine of preparing medicines and ointments. He tried his hand at writing – a short comedy went well, so he attempted something more ambitious and armed with his manuscript he set off to see a literary critic who rejected it and advised Bernard, kindly, to stick to his job. Bernard, however, fancied a change and entered the College de France to read medicine. When he graduated, in 1843, his professor, François Magendie, invited him to become his assistant. On his death in 1858, Bernard succeeded him and also became Professor of Physiology at the Sorbonne.

Bernard had inherited from Magendie the conviction that as animals were part of the natural order of things, they would obey natural laws, and to invoke 'vital spirit' and such like was unnecessary. The task of the physiologist was to study the living organism and search out these laws. Bernard's work is even more remarkable in view of the fact that at the College de France he occupied a dark, damp laboratory in the basement. There was always a chronic shortage of apparatus and he became adept at constructing his own, but it took valuable time from his research. Another difficulty was that he needed animals for his physiology experiments, and was hampered by restrictions imposed by the law. His private life, too, was beset with difficulties, for his wife was violently opposed to his experiments on animals and eventually secured a legal separation.

Some of the extensive experiments Bernard carried out early in his career were on digestion. The accepted view at the time was that digestion took place in the stomach, but Bernard was able to show that a large part of the digestive process took place along the length of the small intestine. Another study he undertook was on the poisonous effect of carbon monoxide. He showed that it had the property of taking the place of oxygen in the blood, causing the body to be deprived of oxygen. He formed the opinion that the red blood cells carried oxygen bound to a chemical. (Some years passed before the chemical was identified). Undoubtedly Bernard had observed that the scarlet colour of oxygenated blood was quite different from the cherry pink colour of the blood with carbon monoxide. In 1851, Bernard, in a series of experiments on the nervous system of rabbits, discovered that the constriction and dilation of blood vessels was under the control of the nervous system. He realised at once that it was the mechanism by which the body controlled the distribution of heat. In a cold environment the surface vessels contracted keeping blood deeper inside the body, whereas in hot surroundings the vessels dilated to enable heat to escape.

Bernard accepted Lavoisier's theory that a process of combustion within the living body was the source of the animal's heat, but he disagreed that the process took place in the lungs. He believed it could not be a direct combustion of carbon in the tissues with oxygen from the air, but an organic process taking place indirectly, perhaps through a series of reactions, and one that took place in all tissues, not just in the lungs. He had been brought to the latter conclusion by an experiment he performed in 1853, in which he compared the temperature in the right and left ventricles of the heart. If Lavoisier was right, it was to be expected that blood within the left ventricle would be at a higher temperature, having just returned, in the pulmonary veins, from the lungs, where Lavoisier believed combustion took place. In fact, Bernard found no temperature difference between them.

In 1856, Bernard found a substance stored in the liver that had been built up from sugar in the blood, and was also capable of being broken down again into sugar. He called it glycogen. He began to see the body as an integrated system, in which a careful balance was kept. When external conditions upset that balance, the body had an inbuilt capacity to right itself. This early idea of homeostasis was a totally new concept in Bernard's day, when the organs and body systems tended to be regarded as independent units. Bernard was a great scientist, honoured by election to the French Academy of Sciences, and given a State funeral.

When the theory of the circulation of the blood was universally accepted, and its function of transporting heat and oxygen round the body established, and blood pressure measurements made, attention turned to the nature of the force driving the blood around. Although 'vital spirit' had been finally exorcised, 'vital force' was now invoked to explain the force that stubbornly resisted explanation in physical terms. Karl Ludwig (1816–95), a German physiologist came along to change all that. In 1847, Ludwig invented the kymograph, that indispensable piece of equipment in the modern physiology laboratory. On the smoked rotating drum, the first continuous recording of blood pressure values was etched. Careful study of the results showed that 'vital force' could go the way of 'vital spirit'; blood circulation was explainable in terms of ordinary mechanical forces. Ludwig was also responsible for showing that gases could be made to evolve from blood exposed to a vacuum, thus making them available for separate study.

About the time Karl Ludwig was born, a French physician, René Laennec (1781–1826), was in the process of inventing a piece of equipment that today's doctors would regard as indispensable. It was the stethoscope. His prototype was nothing more elaborate than a few sheets of paper rolled into a tube and with this he placed one end on the patient's chest and put his ear to the other. As he had hoped, the heart beat and the sound of breathing could be heard quite distinctly. The wooden instrument with which he replaced his paper tube proved to be a valuable aid in the diagnosis of heart and lung diseases. It is ironical that Laennec himself was to die of tuberculosis contracted from a patient in the early days when, conscientious doctor that he was, he would lay his ear close to the patient's chest during his clinical examination. The attempts of doctors like Laennec to correlate a particular set of symptoms with a specific disease was scornfully rejected by a French military doctor, François Broussais (1772–1838), who stated categorically that all diseases were due to inflammation originating in the gut, and the only treatment of value was to bleed the patient. He was an enthusiastic advocate of applying leeches. In 1832, there was an outbreak of cholera, with a high mortality rate, exacerbated by treatment involving bleeding, as recommended by Broussais. He must have been a powerful personality, for in spite of such disasters, he had a considerable following. The demand for leeches increased annually; in 1827, France imported 33 millions, and six years later the figure had risen to 43 millions. Laennec was one of the doctors who fought against the practice, but it took Pierre Louis, a doctor with a talent for statistics, to prove that it was a useless and dangerous practice.

The practice of blood letting was widespread in France long before the time of Broussais. Molière refers to it in *L'Amour Médecin*, 1665. Four doctors are attending the ailing Lucinde, one, Monsieur Tomès, says to Sganarelle, father of Lucinde, 'Sir, we have considered your daughter's illness, and in *my* opinion, it is the result of overheated blood (*grande chaleur de sang*); and so, I recommend bleeding as quickly as you can manage.'

Chapter 9

The Defence Systems of the Blood

While Broussais was leading a campaign in favour of treating all sickness by bleeding, a revolution in medicine was just round the corner. In the third quarter of the 19th century, bacteria, first seen by Leeuwenhoek in the 17th century, were shown to cause disease, and before long new treatments and protective vaccines were being developed.

Matthias Schleiden (1804–1881), a German botanist, made a careful study of plant material under the microscope and found it all composed of small box-like elements, the cells. In some of the cells he could see a central body, the nucleus. He published his findings which were read by Theodor Schwann (1810–82), medically trained assistant to Johannes Müller, a well known German physiologist. Now Schwann liked nothing better than to be allowed to work undisturbed in his little room with his microscope. He had examined countless preparations of animal and human tissues, and he realised that these were also composed of basic elements, the cells. Plants and animals were not so different after all; they were both made up of cells and so there was some fundamental unity of living things. He wondered about the red corpuscles in the blood, were they cells? In 1839, he wrote a book on the structure and growth of plants and animals.

Some years later, on a summer day in 1856, a worried industrialist approached that French chemist of genius, Louis Pasteur (1822–95), with a problem about the production of alcohol by the fermentation of beet juice. Something was going badly wrong and he was at his wit's end to know what to do. The orthodox view at the time was that fermentation, the production of alcohol from sugary liquids, was a purely chemical process. Louis Pasteur was not so sure, in any case he was the last person to worry about orthodoxy in science. Here was a challenge, and a challenge was something he could never resist. Taking samples from healthy vats and sick vats, Pasteur examined them under the microscope. The samples from the healthy vats showed sprouting yeast, and those from the sick vats a mass of rod-like structures. Some scientists who had studied yeast believed it to be a living organism, one had said it sprouted like a plant. During his investigations. Pasteur showed that sugary solutions do not produce alcohol unless yeast is present. He also found that the yeast and the rod-like organisms were destroyed by gentle heat. Pasteur formed the opinion that they were both living organisms – so much for fermentation being a purely chemical process! These micro-organisms were clearly capable of carrying out important chemical reactions.

Seven years later, Napoleon 111 sought Pasteur's help in saving the wine industry. The amount of unpalatable wine being produced had reached almost disastrous proportions. Pasteur investigated the matter and had the answer. When the fermentation is complete, the living organisms must be destroyed by gentle heat before the wine is stored. The vintners found themselves in a dilemma, they faced catastrophe, but to heat the wine would surely ruin it anyway. There was no alternative but to try Pasteur's method – they did so and found it a complete success. It was the first industrial pasteurisation, a process that today we are most likely to associate with milk.

In 1865, Pasteur was again in demand, this time it was trouble in the silk industry. For several years there had been a steady increase in a silkworm disease that was now posing a serious threat to the industry. Could Pasteur help? Pasteur did not know much about silkworms, and it took him six years to complete his research and show that the culprit was a tiny parasite. It was clear to him that the disease was being spread by the handlers and perhaps by the air. He suspected it was caused by a living organism, and simple hygienic measures helped to control it.

Meanwhile, Pasteur was turning over in his mind the process of fermentation, and slowly coming to the conclusion that putrefaction, the breakdown of protein in animal tissue, was also brought about by living organisms. As he saw it, these small living things, the micro-organisms, were probably present in the air and could settle on dead organisms or wounds eating away the flesh and reducing it to a rotting mass. In hospitals the mortality rate following surgery was high. Few operations were performed other than amputations, and the patients were lucky if they escaped the hospital diseases such as septicaemia and gangrene that were so prevalent at the time. Wounds too, readily became infected, often with disastrous results.

Joseph Lister (1827–1912), an English surgeon, read of Pasteur's work and was greatly impressed. The idea that micro-organisms might be responsible for hospital diseases made sense, but how was he to kill them? Pasteur had used heat, but Lister needed an alternative method, and searching in his mind for an idea he recalled having read a paper in which the author had noted that carbolic acid killed parasites in cattle. He decided to try it. During the next few months, after setting all the compound fractures, that is those in which broken bone had penetrated the skin, Lister applied a dressing of carbolic acid. The mortality rate dropped dramatically. Lister published his results in the *Lancet* and wrote to Pasteur. To Pasteur, Lister's results were useful evidence in support of his micro-organism or germ theory of disease. But Pasteur realised that the theory rested on unstable foundations unless he could show conclusively that one distinct kind of micro-organism was associated with a particular disease. Unbeknown to him, another great mind was also at work on the problem.

Robert Koch (1843–1910), was a German doctor whose leanings were towards medical research rather than his country medical practice. As he made his rounds he was constantly reminded of the terrible toll of animal life, and some human life too, taken by the dreaded disease of anthrax. It had been the ruin of many a small farmer, attacking his horses, cattle and sheep. Koch knew all about Pasteur's work, the following he had in France, and that particular germs or bacteria had been found in the blood of animals suffering from anthrax. To Koch, this did not mean that the bacteria were necessarily the cause of the disease. Working in a curtained-off portion of his consulting room, with the most primitive of equipment, Koch developed a technique for isolating particular bacteria. In 1876, he used his own specially made slides containing nutrient liquid and bacteria obtained from an animal with anthrax, which he sealed carefully to prevent contamination, and examined under the microscope. To his delight he was able to watch the bacteria multiply and in time black beads formed, the spores of anthrax. It was a great achievement to culture the bacteria outside the living body. Next, he injected mice with some of the bacteria, they sickened and died. He showed he could inoculate healthy mice with blood from the sick ones and they too would develop anthrax. In this way, passing on the infection from mouse to mouse, he could keep the infection going and still recover the same bacteria after passing through a long chain of mice. Koch had shown that specific bacteria caused a specific disease. His method for establishing the association between specific bacteria and a specific disease is still followed today. Koch postulated that: 'The bacteria must be found in the sick animal, they must be isolated and grown in culture, and when a portion of the culture is inoculated into a healthy animal it must cause the disease. Finally, the same bacteria must be found in the inoculated animal'.

Pasteur, in addition to being a highly creative scientist, was also a great showman who loved an audience. It was he who was able to demonstrate how the disease of anthrax was spread. He showed that anthrax spores were present on the vegetation in pastures, and that they were distributed through the farmers' practice of burying diseased carcases. Earthworms in the soil brought spores from these carcases to the surface in their casts, these dried and were distributed by the wind. Even then, he was able to show, it needed some wound through which bacteria could enter the body. The most minute wound, such as those produced in the mouth when prickly vegetation was consumed, provided a point of entry for these lethal bacteria. Pasteur had a solution to the problem too – burn the carcases and bury the remains deeply.

The quiet, studious and secretive Koch viewed Pasteur, the showman, with a jaundiced eye. He felt that Pasteur had stolen some of his thunder concerning the anthrax, but he had other research under way. He was experimenting with staining bacteria. Looking one day at a blood smear taken from a mouse that had died after being inoculated with putrefying blood, he was surprised to find no bacteria present. Puzzling over the matter, and refusing to believe it, he set about improving the microscope illumination – now something seemed to be present other than the bloodcells, but he could not see clearly what it was. He started again, took a thin smear, dried it and stained it with methyl violet. Success! He could now see masses of minute bacteria. After the most painstaking research, he identified the bacteria responsible for the various infections so prevalent in hospitals at that time. Koch was a master of experimental technique. In 1880 he took up an appointment in the Imperial Health Office in Berlin, where he was provided with two assistants. Up to this time he had been using liquid media for growing bacteria, but trying to separate them in a drop of liquid was an almost impossible task. He progressed to solidifying the media by using agar-agar, that stopped the bacteria moving around so that separate colonies of a single species developed. Pure cultures could be obtained from a colony.

Thus it came about that the germ theory of disease was established. Pasteur's battle cry, 'Look for the microbe!', was taken up. It was now confidently expected that every disease would be shown to have a specific bacterium associated with it, but it was not to prove to be so.

It was well known that animals surviving an attack of anthrax were then immune to the disease. This made Pasteur consider the possibility of achieving immunity in the animals by some artificial means. He had the example of Jenner before him whose technique of vaccination against smallpox had been such an outstanding success. Jenner had made use of the fact that an attack of the mild disease of cowpox gave immunity to smallpox. Unfortunately, there was no such thing as a mild disease associated with anthrax. How could he destroy the virulence of the anthrax bacteria in such a way that they were still capable of producing the disease, but in a mild form? He experimented with heating cultures of the bacteria, and treating them with various chemicals in the hope of producing a suitable vaccine. In 1882, he was confident enough to embark on a public trial of his vaccine. Collecting the large audience he loved, farmers, veterinary surgeons, laboratory staff and other on-lookers, at a farm at Pouilly le Fort, Pasteur had the animals, mostly sheep, with a few goats and cows, separated into two groups. One group was injected with the vaccine. Twelve days later they were given another dose. After a further 14 days, all the animals, vaccinated and untreated, were collected together and given an injection of a virulent strain of anthrax bacteria. Anxious days followed for Pasteur. A few days later some of the vaccinated animals as well as the untreated ones were reported to be sick. Pasteur was worried, he knew his reputation was at stake, but by the time the results were assessed there was no doubt. All the untreated animals were dead and the vaccinated animals were grazing happily, quite unconcerned at the fate of their fellows.

Pasteur was to go on to produce a vaccine against rabies. Koch was to isolate the bacterium of tuberculosis. Now, thanks to these two great men, techniques were available for isolating bacteria, and rules established for identifying the causative agent of a disease. The possibility of producing vaccines against other diseases had been opened up.

But no one yet knew anything about the mechanism of immunity. In Berlin, in 1884, one of Koch's assistants, Friedrich Löeffler (1852–1915), isolated the diphtheria bacillus. In Paris, workers in Pasteur's laboratory had discovered that diphtheria bacteria were confined to the throat. If the infection was localised, why did the disease have such a high mortality rate? They isolated and cultured the bacteria, then filtered them off from the culture solution. To their surprise, they found that the filtrate, which was free of bacteria, was highly poisonous to animals. This explained why, although the bacteria were localised, the disease was so deadly – a poisonous material, a toxin, was produced by the bacteria. Work began in an attempt to find a vaccine.

A similar effort was being made in Koch's laboratory in Berlin. Emil Behring (1854–1917), was a German, born of a poorish family, he studied at the Friedrich Wilhelms Institute in Berlin where he received a free education in medicine in return for 10 years army service as a military surgeon. The possibility of combating infectious disease by the use of disinfectants was of great interest to him. Iodoform came into use for the treatment of wounds at about this time and he was to make use of the chemical later, in his research. In 1889, at the end of his service, he became assistant to Koch, at the Institute for Hygiene, at the University of Berlin. Behring decided to investigate the effect of iodoform on different bacteria, he had in mind an idea that it might be possible to find a systemic disinfecting agent. The early results were encouraging. He experimented with other iodine compounds on cultures of diphtheria bacteria, evaluating their effectiveness by inoculating guinea pigs with portions of the treated culture. Most still developed the disease and succumbed, a few survived. The surviving animals were immune to further doses of diptheria bacteria. That animals surviving a particular disease bacame immune was not news – it had already been shown to be true for smallpox, anthrax and other diseases. Behring was determined to find out what actually happened to bring about this immunity. He was sure that there must be some changes taking place in the blood. Surely some substance must be formed and remain in circulation while the immunity lasted, perhaps for life?

In his next round of experiments, Behring drew some blood from an immune animal, and after allowing it to clot, took a little of the serum that separated from it and mixed it with some of the culture of diphtheria bacteria. He then injected the mixture into an untreated guinea pig. Using a second guinea pig as a control, he injected it with some of the same culture of diphtheria bacteria without the serum. The first guinea pig remained healthy, the second developed the disease and died. Behring's hunch had paid off – something in the serum had prevented the diphtheria bacteria from producing the toxin. The emphasis of his research now shifted from the idea of a systemic disinfectant to the use of blood serum. Next, he tried the effect of an injection of the serum on animals already infected with diphtheria toxin. The animals improved and recovered. Behring had prepared an antitoxin, a serum capable of neutralising the effects of a toxin. It was the first antitoxin, and the result of a first class piece of research. A colleague of Behring's was the Japanese bacteriologist, Shibasaburo Kitasato (1856–1931), who isolated the tetanus bacillus and showed that like diphtheria, it was the toxin produced that was the dangerous material.

Independently, Pasteur's laboratory prepared a diphtheria antitoxin by the immunisation of horses, a procedure that Behring later adopted. The work of the German and French pioneers was to lay the foundations for the control of many diseases of man and animals. In many ways the work of Pasteur and Koch was complementary, but an intense nationalistic rivalry always existed between them, indeed it may well have spurred them on to greater efforts.

It was the accepted practice in Pasteur's laboratory that no scientist should gain financially from his discoveries, but in Koch's laboratory there was no such code of practice. Behring patented his diphtheria antitoxin and reaped many rewards both financially and in terms of prestige. In 1895, he was appointed Director of the Institute of Hygiene, in Marburg. Within a few years he decided that his next task was to fight tuberculosis. He was never able to prepare a vaccine, but much of importance came from his work. For example, he discovered that children could contract tuberculosis by drinking milk infected with the bacteria of bovine tuberculosis. It drew attention to the importance of disease in cattle. In 1901, Behring was honoured by his country and became entitled to call himself von Behring. In the same year he received the Nobel Prize in medicine, the first to be awarded. In 1913, Behring had developed a preventive vaccine against diphtheria, a toxin and antitoxin mixture stabilised by formaldehyde.

Paul Ehrlich (1854–1915), another of Koch's scientists, contributed to Behring's work on diphtheria antitoxin. Ehrlich studied in Breslau and Strasburg, graduating in medicine in 1877. He was particularly interested in chemistry during his student days, and fascinated by the use of chemical dyes in microscope technique. He tried out various combinations of dyes on animal and plant tissues and observed the different effects of acidic and basic stains. He joined the staff of the medical clinic in the Charité Hospital in Berlin, becoming head physician, and later, in 1884, professor. While at the hospital, he found he could distinguish between a number of blood diseases by examining blood cells in his stained preparations. This gave him the idea that chemical affinities controlled biological processes. He also estimated the number of red blood cells in one cubic centimetre of blood and noted different types of white blood cells shown up by his staining technique. He even tried out methylene blue as a treatment for malaria when he discovered that it stained the parasites. While he was there he was unfortunate enough to contract tuberculosis, thus necessitating a prolonged convalescence in the warm dry climate of Egypt. When he returned to Berlin two years later, he set up a small laboratory of his own.

In his private laboratory, Ehrlich investigated immune reactions in mice. He fed small quantities of toxic plant proteins, ricin and abrin, to mice, gradually increasing the dose. Serum from these actively immunised mice, when injected into untreated mice, conferred on them a passive immunity and protected them from the poisonous effect of the plant proteins. Furthermore, litters bred from the immunised mice were found to possess a short-lived immunity, sustained by suckling from the immunised mother. Ehrlich also found that a litter from a non-immunised mother could be protected by suckling from an immunised mother. Koch heard of his work and invited him to join the staff of the newly formed Institute for Infectious Diseases in Berlin. It is said of Ehrlich that he conducted his research in a cloud of cigar smoke and wrote notes on his cuffs, but true or false, there is no doubt that he had an exceptionally able and creative mind.

While he was at Koch's Institute, Ehrlich continued to work on toxins and antitoxins, and assisted Behring to produce a potent diphtheria antitoxin. By immunising large animals, Behring and Ehrlich were able to produce sufficient antitoxin for concentration, purification and use in clinical trials. In 1894, diphtheria antitoxin was given to 220 children with the disease, with marked success. It was discovered that large initial doses gave the best results. By 1895, antitoxin development was going so well that control laboratories were needed and a new Institute for the investigation and control of sera was opened in a Berlin suburb, with Ehrlich as director. It was no elegant new building but was housed in a disused bakery. Ehrlich's laboratory was grossly overcrowded, but he saw only those items of immediate concern, and thus, in his single-mindedness, the clutter of used equipment, notes and papers were invisible to him as he wove his way around his littered laboratory. His aim was to standardise the antitoxin, describe the potency in terms of international units of antitoxin, and distribute the material in dried form and vacuum packed.

In 1906, a new building was opened for the Institute. With an increased staff Ehrlich was able to investigate a theory he held that chemical compounds could be used to cure a disease, not just alleviate the symptoms. He imagined the possibility of chemical compounds seeking out and destroying micro-organisms in the body. He called such compounds 'magic bullets'. In 1908, before the most important work of his life got under way, Ehrlich was awarded the Nobel Prize for medicine, jointly with Mechnikov (whom we shall meet shortly), for work on immunity. Ehrlich's first success in this direction was the use of trypan red to kill trypanosomes (protozoa) in infected mice, but to his disappointment he found it was ineffective against the parasites causing sleeping sickness in humans. Nevertheless, there was an arsenical compound, atoxyl, that had given promising results in the treatment of sleeping sickness, and Ehrlich believed that more effective derivatives of atoxyl could be made. The accepted formula of this substance was basically a benzene ring with a single side chain. If correct, it would not be expected to form stable derivatives, but

Ehrlich was convinced it had two side chains, and if *that* was correct it *would* form stable derivatives. Ehrlich proved to be right. He and his staff prepared nearly a thousand, each meticulously tested on animals. Compound number 606 was effective against the spirochaetes (a type of bacterium), causing syphilis, the most serious of the venereal diseases. Effective, yes, but how safe? Ehrlich had to find the answer. Two members of his staff volunteered to try it on themselves. No harm resulted. In 1910, Ehrlich announced the discovery of 'Salvarsan', the 606th derivative. Ehrlich had opened up a new field, the study of chemotherapy.

In 1882, Ilya Mechnikov (1845–1916), was carrying out some research on marine organisms in the Mediterranean, off the coast of Sicily. It was the same year that Pasteur was demonstrating the value of his anthrax vaccine at Pouilly le Fort, and Ehrlich was working at the Charité Hospital in Berlin, examining patients' blood smears under the microscope. Mechnikov was born in Kharkov, in Russia, and had ambitions to study medicine, but was diverted to zoology. He was a temperamental and eccentric man who twice attempted to commit suicide. He studied first at Kharkov and later at universities in Germany, and spent some time working at the biological stations in Heligoland and Naples before being appointed professor at the University of Odessa. In 1882, inheritances made him financially independent and off he went to Messina, in Italy, where he took a great delight in anatomical and physiological studies of invertebrates, becoming an authority on the marine fauna of the Sicilian coast.

Mechnikov was particularly interested in digestion. One day, he was examining the transparent larvae of starfish under the microscope when he noticed mobile cells inside. Careful observation showed that during the process of metamorphosis of the larvae the mobile cells re-absorbed those parts of the larvae no longer required. He discovered that these mobile cells were not derived from the endoderm, the layer that gives rise to the digestive system, but from the mesoderm. This odd fact lay dormant in his mind for some time. On another occasion, he watched minute particles in the body fluid of a sea urchin being ingested by the amoeba-like activity of some cells. He had a flash of inspiration. Could cells like these defend the organism against invaders such as bacteria, by engulfing them? He had to calm himself in order to organise his thoughts. Still enthusiastic about his new idea, Mechnikov collected some small thorns and inserted them carefully into the starfish larvae. What would happen? He could scarcely wait for the results of his experiment. Very early next morning he was delighted to find that mobile cells had assembled and surrounded the thorns. Next, he inoculated the larvae with bacteria and watched as mobile cells gathered and surrounded them. His third experiment was on the water flea, Daphnia; through its transparent body he could see the blood cells, and when yeast cells invaded the body they assembled on the scene (yeast sometimes invades Daphnia and grows inside the body, destroying it).

Mechnikov found all this very promising and he decided to see if anything similar occurred in higher animals. Eventually he was able to demonstrate that white blood cells, derived from the mesoderm of the embryo, were capable of ingesting bacteria. He called these white cells in mammalian blood, 'phagocytes'. Any injury or infection alerted the phagocytes and brought them hurrying to the site, their activity causing inflammation. When there was a big battle, the degenerating bodies of phagocytes and invaders formed the pus. Mechnikov was convinced that phagocytes were an important factor in the body's defence system. It was totally in opposition to the accepted theory of the time, which was that the white blood cells made a suitable environment for the growth of bacteria. Mechnikov was certain he was on the right track, in his mind he had already moved on to more important questions. If phagocytes ingested bacteria and prevented disease, why did the system fail sometimes, allowing the disease to develop? Why did the immunised and untreated animals behave differently when virulent bacteria were injected? He believed the white blood cells in the immunised animals had become 'trained' in some way and were all ready when bacteria entered the body. Mechnikov published the work he had done, but as so often happened with a brilliant new idea, no one took very much notice. In 1886, he was invited back to Odessa, where a new bacteriological institute had been established; he went, but he was unhappy with the general disharmony. In spite of his depression he had faith in his phagocyte theory, and in 1887, he set off to visit Koch and Pasteur. Koch rejected Mechnikov's ideas but Pasteur felt that the young man might be on to something important. He already had quite a lot of published work to his credit, and he invited Mechnikov to join his laboratory. Mechnikov settled there and remained for the rest of his life, becoming very much respected and admired by all.

Another problem of particular interest to Mechnikov, was the reason for the arrival and departure of epidemics, especially cholera. He agreed with Pettenkofer, Professor of Hygiene at the University of Munich, that for an epidemic to arise, something more than the disease organism itself was necessary. Pettenkofer, however, refused to accept the germ theory of disease at all, and to show his contempt for it, he swallowed a fresh culture of cholera bacteria, much to the horror of his students. Astonishingly, he did not develop the disease. What had protected him? Mechnikov decided to repeat the experiment. As always he observed his reactions with scientific detachment. No disease resulted! However, a third experiment, carried out by a student of Mechnikov's, resulted in the young man becoming desperately ill and almost losing his life. The mystery of epidemics remained unexplained.

When Pasteur died, in 1895, Mechnikov succeeded him as Director of the Institute. In 1908, he shared with Paul Ehrlich the Nobel Prize for medicine, for their research on immunity.

Chapter 10

The Discovery of the Blood Groups

Attempts at blood transfusion had been made at least as early as the 17th century, sometimes they were successful, sometimes they were a complete disaster. The reason for these hitherto inexplicable results was discovered by the Austrian-born immunologist, Karl Landsteiner (1868–1943). Landsteiner was trained in medicine at the University of Vienna. He was a modest man, well read, musical and an excellent pianist. His early work was in chemistry, but by 1897, he was assistant to the Director of the Pathological Anatomical Institute in Vienna, where, during his stay, he performed over 3,500 post mortems. Eventually, by 1919, the poor working conditions had got him down and he moved to The Hague, in Holland, taking up an appointment at the RK Hospital. He did not find conditions there much better, so he made up his mind to go to the USA. There, in 1922, he joined the Rockefeller Institute, in New York, and by 1929, he had become an American citizen.

Landsteiner published his first paper in 1900, and in a footnote gave the first information on agglutination, the clumping together of red blood cells from some individuals when mixed with the serum of another. He attributed this reaction to individual differences. For 40 years blood reactions were to be a major subject of his investigations, but other important work was to be conducted in his laboratory, notably research on syphilis, poliomyelitis and typhus.

Following up his observation on agglutination, he set about separating whole blood into red blood cells and serum. Testing suspensions of red blood cells against different sera, he found that, on the basis of whether or not agglutination occurred, he could divide whole blood into three groups; A, B and O. The red blood cells themselves belonged to three groups; A, B and O, and the sera to two groups, anti-A and anti-B. Two of Landsteiner's assistants, Decastello and Sturli, found a fourth whole-blood group, AB. The results of the tests may be summarised in a table,

Blood group	Serum anti-A	Serum anti-B
A	+	−
B	−	+
AB	+	+
O	−	−

+ = agglutination
− = no agglutination

Figure 4 The results of ABO blood grouping tests.

Landsteiner believed that the red blood cells bore antigens. An individual had antigens, A, B, both or neither, and his serum had the antibodies, anti-A, anti-B, both or neither. The A antigen in the red blood cells, he believed, gave rise to agglutination when the cells were mixed with serum containing anti-A antibodies, therefore, they were never found together in the same individual. Likewise, the B antigen and anti-B serum were not found together. Where both antigens A and B occurred, no antibodies of the anti-A or anti-B type were present; and where neither the A nor B antigen existed, both anti-A and anti-B antibodies were present in the serum. (The reader may wonder why the presence of one or more antigens in the red blood cells does not stimulate the production of the corresponding antibody. An individual's antigens, present before the first few months of life when the ability to produce antibodies is developed, do not normally stimulate the production of antibodies.)

To determine the ABO blood group to which an individual belongs, a few cubic centimetres of fresh blood are allowed to clot in a narrow test tube, and the serum removed. Part of the clot is stirred with a 0.9% sodium

Blood group	Antigens on red cells	Antibodies in serum
A	A	Anti-B
B	B	Anti-A
AB	A+B	None
O	O	Anti-A + Anti-B

Figure 5 Antigens and antibodies in the ABO blood group system.

chloride solution, centrifuged, and the cells re-suspended in fresh solution to make a 2–3% suspension of packed cells. Two drops of the suspension are now added to each of three tubes, the first containing one drop of anti-A serum, the second one drop of anti-B serum, and the third one drop of serum containing anti-A and anti-B. The tubes are shaken and left at 20–25°C for two hours, then examined for agglutination.

Here then, was the necessary theoretical basis for a transfusion of compatible blood, but several years passed before much practical use was made of it, for other problems remained, notably the clotting of blood when in contact with the air.

In 1910, following the rediscovery of Mendel's laws of inheritance some ten years earlier, Von Dungern and Hirszfeld put forward a hypothesis for the inheritance of blood groups. In 1924, Bernstein, a mathematician, made some amendments to it and a theory was established. The ABO blood group system consists of three alternative forms (alleles) of a single gene. A and B are equally dominant (co-dominants) to O, which is recessive. One form of the gene will be derived from each parent, either A, B or O, therefore six combinations are possible in the individual; AA, AO, BB, BO, AB, and OO. The antigens A and B are present on the red cells and when blood of an unknown group is tested with anti-A and anti-B sera, AA and AO cannot be distinguished, and neither can BB and BO. Accordingly, only four groups can be identified by this means; A, B, AB, and O.

In 1914, Richard Lewisohn showed that the addition of citrates to blood prevented coagulation, and at about the same time it was found to be possible to store blood under refrigeration for a period of two to three weeks. However, the blood transfusion service was not set up until 1939, when technical advances together with experience gained during the Spanish Civil War made it a practical proposition. Blood transfusion then became much more widely practised and has been responsible for the saving of countless lives. Prospects for operating on the heart, lungs and circulatory system now began to look brighter, and with the development of the heart-lung machine, a piece of apparatus that can oxygenate and pump around the patient's blood, the era of open heart surgery arrived.

When a volunteer donates blood, his blood group is determined, then, using sterilised equipment, about 400 cm^3 of blood from a vein in his arm is drawn into a bottle containing sodium citrate to prevent clotting. Meanwhile, before a patient receives a transfusion, not only will his blood group be checked, but an additional compatibility test will be carried out between his blood and that of the donor. Two drops of a suspension of the donor's red cells in saline solution are mixed with two drops of the patient's serum. It is centrifuged or incubated and examined for agglutination. This test is an additional check on any possibility of error or rare anomalous agglutinations. After the test has been performed, the blood, at the correct temperature and carefully regulated rate, is fed into a vein in the patient's arm.

In 1926, Landsteiner and Levine discovered that there were sub-groups of group A, and in the following year, they found that human red cells bore other antigens, M, N and P. However, they were of no importance in blood transfusion as human serum does not contain the corresponding antibodies.

In 1940, Landsteiner, Weiner and Levine injected blood from a Rhesus monkey into rabbits and guinea pigs. The small animals would then be expected to produce antibodies against the antigens present in the red blood cells of the Rhesus monkey. From the blood of the rabbits and guinea pigs they prepared a serum by removing the blood cells. This serum not only agglutinated the red cells of the Rhesus monkey, but was found to bring about agglutination of the red cells in many samples of human blood taken from the white population in New York. Agglutination, in fact, was calculated to occur in 85% of the population. The red blood cells of such people have the Rhesus antigen and are said to be Rhesus positive (Rh positive or Rh+, for short), that of the remaining 15%, in which no agglutination takes place, lack the Rhesus antigen and are said to be Rhesus negative (Rh negative or Rh-, for short). The Rhesus antigen may be associated with the red cells of any of the four ABO blood groups. Inheritance was believed to depend upon a gene with only two alleles. (The situation has since been found to be much more complex, but it need not concern us here.) Taking the alleles as R (dominant) and r (recessive), Rhesus positive individuals have a genetic make-up (genotype), RR or Rr, and Rhesus negative individuals, rr. A child will inherit one gene, R or r, from each parent. Where the parents are both Rhesus negative, rr, the child will clearly be the same; where they are both Rhesus positive, RR, or one is RR and the other Rr, the child will be Rhesus positive, but a child of parents both Rr, stands a 25% chance of being Rhesus negative. The following diagram may help to make this clear.

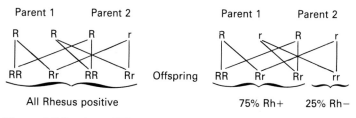

Figure 6 Offspring of Rh+ parents bearing Rh- genes.

Later, as further blood sub-groups were discovered, Landsteiner believed that an individual's blood would be shown to be as unique as a fingerprint – a 'serological fingerprint', in fact.

Following the discovery of the Rhesus factor, Levine came to the conclusion that it was involved in the haemolytic disease of the new-born (erythroblastosis foetalis), the symptoms of which are anaemia and jaundice. He noticed that most babies with the disease were Rhesus positive and their mothers Rhesus negative.

Although the Rhesus antigen is present in 85% of the population, the corresponding antibody is produced only under special conditions. One way in which this could take place is if a Rhesus negative person were to receive a transfusion of blood of the correct ABO group, but of the Rhesus positive type. Under these conditions the anti-Rhesus antibodies will be produced in the blood of the recipient. Little harm results at this stage, but if a second transfusion of Rhesus positive blood were to be given at a later date, the anti-Rhesus antibodies, already present in the recipient's blood would result in agglutination of the donor's red blood cells, causing blockage of the blood vessels. As there was a gap of 30 years between the discovery of the ABO groups and the Rhesus factor, things went wrong occasionally. The second way in which anti-Rhesus antibodies may arise, is when a Rhesus negative woman married to a Rhesus positive man, is pregnant with a Rhesus positive foetus. There is a possibility that blood cells from the foetus may enter the maternal circulation through leakage at the placenta during delivery. If this occurs, the Rhesus antigens on the foetal red cells will bring about production of anti-Rhesus antibodies in the maternal blood, these will not affect her red blood cells as she lacks the antigen, but they will remain in the circulation. In any subsequent pregnancy with another Rhesus positive foetus, anti-Rhesus antibodies may reach the foetal circulation and react with the red blood cells. In severe cases the child may be stillborn, otherwise it may be anaemic and jaundiced to some degree, suffering from erythroblastosis foetalis, as Levine noticed. Treatment, after blood transfusion techniques had been perfected, consisted of replacing the affected blood of the newly-born child, with fresh blood.

Today, if an expectant mother is found to be Rhesus negative, the husband's blood is also tested. If he proves to be Rhesus positive, prophylactic measures are taken to suppress the production of anti-Rhesus antibodies in the mother. Another precaution taken is to ensure that Rhesus negative women of childbearing age are never given blood transfusions of Rhesus positive blood, in case they become sensitised and produce anti-Rhesus antibodies. There is no problem in the case of a Rhesus positive mother carrying a Rhesus negative foetus, for the antibody mechanism of a child does not begin to function until it is several months old.

To return to the problem of the Rhesus negative mother with the Rhesus positive foetus: in Britain, the risk of erythroblastosis foetalis is only about 0.6%, even though 15% of women are Rhesus negative. A number of factors operate to limit the risk; first babies are not affected, the husband may be Rhesus negative and therefore the child will be Rhesus negative also, leakage through the placenta may be insufficient to stimulate the production of anti-Rhesus antibodies, and in any case, some women do not respond to the introduction of Rhesus positive red cells by producing the appropriate antibody. A particularly interesting situation occurs when the mother is Group O, Rhesus negative. If the baby is Group A, Rhesus positive and the red cells from the baby leak into the maternal circulation at delivery, they are destroyed by the anti-A antibodies present in the plasma of the Group O mother, before they have time to stimulate the production of anti-Rhesus antibodies. A similar reaction occurs if the baby is Group B, Rhesus positive, as the maternal Group O blood also contains anti-B antibodies. Where the baby is Group AB, Rhesus positive, its red cells will also be destroyed by the maternal antibodies.

If this is Nature's way of dealing with the problem, why not give anti-Rhesus antibodies to the Rhesus negative mother at risk, following delivery of her first baby? The idea was suggested to Cyril Clarke, Professor of Medicine at the University of Liverpool. Clarke was born in 1907, and was educated at Cambridge, where he received a doctorate in science, and at Guy's Hospital where he obtained his medical qualifications. During the 1939–45 war, he served with the RNVR. In addition to occupying the Chair of Medicine at Liverpool, he was Director of the Nuffield Unit of Medical Genetics at Liverpool, and consultant physician to the United Liverpool Hospitals. He was President of the Royal College of Physicians from 1972–77, and is the author of a number of textbooks and papers in scientific journals. He has been in great demand as a lecturer and committee member, and he was awarded the CBE in 1969, elected to the Royal Society in 1970 and knighted in 1974. Clarke considered the suggestion carefully. At first, to provide the mother's blood with anti-Rhesus antibodies appeared to be the very thing to avoid. But perhaps injected anti-Rhesus antibodies might react with the Rhesus positive cells from the child before they could cause trouble?

The first experiments carried out by Clarke and his colleagues involved male volunteers. They each received an injection of Rhesus positive red blood cells labelled with radioactive chromium atoms. Half the volunteers were then given an injection of anti-Rhesus antibodies. At first, the results appeared promising, a high proportion of the Rhesus positive cells were destroyed, but after six months it was found that anti-Rhesus antibodies had built up in the blood. The problem appeared to be that although the anti-Rhesus antibodies destroyed the Rhesus positive cells, their residues still behaved as antigens. A second series of experiments was carried out using an 'incomplete' anti-Rhesus antibody that appears to coat the antigen in such a way that it does not provoke the antibody-producing cells to react. These experiments were more successful, production of anti-Rhesus antibodies was suppressed in most of the volunteers.

The production of anti-Rhesus antibodies in the bloodstream of a Rhesus negative mother following delivery of the first Rhesus positive child is related to the amount of red blood cells received from the child. Therefore, for their first clinical trials, Clarke and his co-workers selected mothers from whom blood smears showed they had received a fair number of foetal red cells. (The smear is prepared by a special technique that removes haemoglobin from the maternal red cells but not from those of the foetus, leaving the latter readily seen under the microscope.) They injected a preparation consisting of anti-Rhesus gamma globulin instead of the anti-Rhesus serum previously used, a preparation that avoids any possible risk of jaundice. It had been prepared from the serum of the immunised male volunteers. The injection was given to 131 mothers at risk within 48 hours of delivery. Six months later only one had produced the anti-Rhesus antibodies in the blood. A control group of 136 mothers showed that after six months 21 had anti-Rhesus antibodies in the blood. Any fears that a mother might produce the antibodies following a second similar pregnancy have proved unfounded.

In addition to his work on blood groups, Landsteiner and Finger showed, in 1906, while Landsteiner was still in Vienna, that they were able to explain the mechanism of the Wasserman reaction, a test for syphilis. It involved testing for the presence of the antibody produced by the syphilous patient, by means of the antigen. In 1907, Landsteiner found that the antigen, previously extracted from human organs infected with syphilis, could be replaced by an extract prepared from ox heart.

Between 1908 and 1922, Landsteiner was also researching on poliomyelitis. He injected a preparation of brain and spinal cord, obtained from a victim of the disease, into a Rhesus monkey, it developed paralysis. Landsteiner could find no bacteria in the nervous system and he concluded, quite correctly, that a virus must be responsible. In collaboration with Levaditi of the Pasteur Institute, in Paris, he developed a procedure for the diagnosis of poliomyelitis. Yet another success from Landsteiner's laboratory, was his discovery with Nigg, in 1930–32, that *Rickettsia prowazeki*, the organism causing typhus could be cultured on living media. This greatly facilitated work on the disease.

In 1930, Landsteiner received the Nobel Prize for medicine. The discovery of the blood groups was to have far more than clinical significance, as important as that was. The techniques for the identification of blood groups was to provide a new tool in the hands of researchers outside the medical field, as will be seen in a later chapter.

Chapter 11

Exploring the Biochemistry of Blood

In the mid-19th century, Claude Bernard had come to the conclusion that red blood cells carried oxygen bound to a chemical. In 1862, Ernst Seyler (1825–95), a German biochemist, isolated a mysterious crystalline substance from red blood cells – it was named haemoglobin. Haemoglobin was found to be largely protein in nature, and accounted for 95% of the total protein in red blood cells. Haemoglobin is in fact a protein, globin, attached to a non-protein part containing iron, called haem. The chemical structure of haem was elucidated, atom by atom, by the great German organic chemist, Hans Fischer (1881–1945), Professor of Chemistry in the University of Munich. He confirmed his analysis of haem by synthesising it in 1929, a remarkable accomplishment for which he was awarded the Nobel Prize in chemistry in the following year. The analysis of globin was to take longer.

Proteins are colloids, giant molecules that remain suspended in solution because they are continually punched around by water molecules. Theodor Svedberg (1884–1971), Professor of Physical Chemistry at the University of Uppsala, in Sweden, had the idea that protein molecules might be persuaded to settle out if an effect equivalent to many times that of the force of gravity at the earth's surface could be developed. Such an effect is produced in the centrifuge. Centrifuges were already in use that could separate relatively large particles from the liquid in which they were suspended, such as blood cells from the plasma, but to separate the very much smaller colloid particles was another problem. Svedberg developed the ultracentrifuge, capable of spinning the material round so fast that it produced an effect equivalent to hundreds of thousands of times that of normal gravity. The giant molecules of protein obligingly settled out in the ultracentrifuge, and moreover, they settled at different rates from the mixture, making some separation possible. The rate at which each separated could be used to calculate the molecular mass. For his work on colloids, Svedberg received the Nobel Prize for chemistry, in 1926.

Extracts from living tissues usually contain an assortment of proteins, often closely related, and the separation of them posed a problem. Arne Tiselius (1902–1971), was born in Stockholm and educated at the University of Uppsala where he was a student of Svedberg's. After he gained his doctorate in 1928, he became Svedberg's assistant, and ten years later he was Professor of Biochemistry. Tiselius took up an observation made in 1899 by Sir William Hardy, an English biologist, that protein molecule in colloidal solution has a pattern of positive and negative electric charges distributed on it and it will therefore behave in a particular way in an electric field. When the charges are added up they may leave a positive or a negative charge or possibly no charge at all. No two patterns of charge are identical, and therefore the behaviour in an electric field will be different. If a solution of different proteins is taken and an electric current passed through it, some of the proteins will travel towards one electrode, some towards the other, all at different rates, and thus they will become separated. The process is electrophoresis. That sounded fine in theory but it did not become a practical proposition until Tiselius, using a jelly-like medium and a piece of specially designed apparatus, began to work on the problem. The ingenious piece of apparatus that Tiselius designed consisted of a set of tubes that could be fixed together, by means of ground glass joints, into a ⌐⎯⎯⌐ shape. By taking the tube apart, different proteins could be collected from the separate sections. Tiselius was able to follow the progress of the separation by using special lenses to observe changes in the refractive index, that is, changes in the bending of the light rays passing through the suspension. Changes in the refractive index could be recorded photographically and used as a basis for calculating the quantity of each protein present. If electrophoresis of protein failed to separate individual proteins, the protein preparation was, in all probability, pure. In 1938, Tiselius was appointed Director of the Institute of Biochemistry in Stockholm, and in 1948 he was awarded the Nobel Prize in chemistry, for his work on the technique of separating proteins.

Cohn investigated the proteins of blood plasma by electrophoresis and chemical methods, and found that albumin, a water soluble protein, accounted for half of these proteins, and that about 35% of them were made up of larger molecules, globulins. Globulins are insoluble in water but soluble in dilute salt solution. Cohn found they could be divided into three fractions; alpha, beta and gamma. Gamma-globulins have been found to be important in the immune system.

Frederick Sanger, an English biochemist, born in 1918, and educated at the University of Cambridge, laboured in the Medical Research Council's Laboratory of Molecular Biology at Cambridge, to elucidate the structure of protein molecules. It was already known that they could be broken down into smaller molecules, polypeptides, and that these in turn could be shown to be built up from amino acids. There are over twenty different amino acids, so in a particular protein the problems were: Which amino acids are present? In what order are the amino acids linked in the molecular chain? In 1945, Sanger began by breaking the protein molecule in such a way that small chains of amino acids were obtained. This may be done by means of an enzyme. Sanger discovered that a chemical, 2:4 dinitrofluorobenzene (later known as Sanger's Reagent), would attach itself to one end of the short chain of amino acids but not the other. Further enzyme action was then harnessed to break down the chain into its constituent amino acids. Sanger now needed a method of separating the amino acids, in order to find out which one was attached to his reagent, for that was the one at the vulnerable end of the chain. A new technique was at hand, it was paper chromatography, developed by Martin and Synge, in 1944. They were also Nobel Prizewinners in chemistry, for the year 1952. The field of protein chemistry is notable for its number of Nobel Laureates.

The technique of paper chromatography consists of placing a small concentrated spot of the amino acid mixture to be analysed, near the lower edge of a strip of filter paper, and allowing it to dry. The strip is then placed with the lower edge in a suitable solvent mixture. As the solvent creeps up the paper by capillarity, the amino acids also creep up with the solvent, but at varying rates owing to their different solubilities in the solvent. Eventually, the amino acids become separated. Various tests are available for identifying them, and the chromatogram may be matched against chromatograms obtained for known amino acids.

Sanger applied his method of analysing proteins particularly to the investigation of the structure of insulin (a hormone found in the pancreas of animals and used in the treatment of diabetes). By 1953 after eight years of elegant research, he had elucidated the structure. It was the first protein to have the sequence of amino acids along the polypeptide chain resolved. In 1958, Sanger received the Nobel Prize in chemistry. Six years later, insulin had been synthesised. In 1980, Sanger received the Nobel Prize in chemistry for the second time, sharing it with Gilbert and Berg, for their work on nucleic acids. Following Sanger's great success with insulin, the sequence of amino acid units in other proteins was worked out, including that in myoglobin, by Edmundson and Hirs, in 1961, and in haemoglobin by Schroeder, in 1963.

Max Perutz and John Kendrew of the Medical Research Council's Unit for Molecular Biology, at Cambridge, undertook the task of elucidating the three-dimensional structure of the protein molecules, myoglobin and haemoglobin. Perutz worked principally on haemoglobin, Kendrew on myoglobin.

John Kendrew was born in 1917, and educated at the Universities of Bristol and Cambridge. During the 1939–45 war he worked in the Ministry of Aircraft Production. From

1946–75, he was Deputy Director of the Medical Research Council's Unit for Molecular Biology at Cambridge. He has held many important positions, including membership of the Council for Scientific Policy (1965–72), Secretary General of the European Molecular Biology Conference (1969–72), President of the International Union for Pure and Applied Biophysics (1969–72), and Secretary General of the International Council for Scientific Unions (1974–80). He was elected a Fellow of the Royal Society in 1960, and awarded the Nobel Prize for chemistry jointly with Perutz, in 1962. In the following year he was awarded the CBE, and in 1974 he was knighted. Kendrew has edited the Journal of Molecular Biology since 1959. At present he is Director General of the European Molecular Biology Laboratory in Heidelberg, an appointment he took up in 1975.

Myoglobin is found in muscle tissue. Its task is to pick up oxygen released by the red blood cells, store it, and transfer it to energy-producing bodies, the mitochondria, in the cells where glucose is combined with oxygen to form carbon dioxide and water, with the release of energy – the process of cell respiration. When Kendrew set to work on myoglobin, it was known to consist of a single polypeptide chain of about 150 amino acid units attached to a haem group. Although methods of determining the nature of the units and the order in which they were linked already existed, it told only part of the story, for the 150 amino acid units were capable of an almost infinite number of spatial arrangements. It was discovering the precise arrangement they held that constituted the challenge to Kendrew. It had already been discovered that side chains form cross links in proteins thus folding the molecule into an approximately spherical shape – the shape of most protein molecules. By cross links certain amino acids are brought together folding the molecule into a particular shape or configuration, forming the 'active site' of the molecule where it fits a complementary 'active site' in another molecule as it undergoes a chemical reaction.

Many proteins form crystals. The fact that they crystallise means that they are capable of forming a regular three-dimensional arrangement of identical molecules. The best technique for studying crystals is X-ray crystallography. X-rays are electromagnetic waves of very short wavelength. The crystal is studied by turning it while a beam of X-rays is directed through it. The rays produce a central spot on a photographic film and a pattern of fainter spots around it – the X-ray diffraction pattern. The pattern is caused by the X-rays being scattered or deflected by the electrons in the outer part of each atom in the crystal. Crystals of different composition have different and characteristic X-ray diffraction patterns. If the structure of a crystal is known, its X-ray diffraction pattern can be worked out. The process can be operated in reverse, but myoglobin, although by comparison with other proteins a small molecule, nevertheless contains about 2,500 atoms. It presented a formidable task until, in 1953, an important discovery made by Max Perutz, provided the key that eventually made it possible.

Max Perutz was born in Vienna, in 1914. He left the University of Vienna in 1936, after the Nazi power in Germany became an increasing threat to his country, and continued his studies at the University of Cambridge, where he gained his Ph.D in X-ray crystallography in 1940. From 1939–45, he was assistant to William Bragg, a renowned physicist and youngest-ever Nobel Laureate. Such was Perutz's success that in 1947, he was appointed Director of the Medical Research Council's Unit for Molecular Biology, a position he occupied until 1962, when the Medical Research Council built the Laboratory of Molecular Biology for him and his team. He continued as Director until 1979. He has served in a number of other important capacities: Chairman of the European Molecular Biology organisation (1963–69), Reader at the Davy Faraday Research Laboratory at the Royal Institution (1954–68), and Fullerian Professor of Physiology (1973–79). Perutz was elected a Fellow of the Royal Society in 1954, and became a Companion of Honour in 1975. With Kendrew he shared the Nobel Prize in chemistry, in 1962. Perutz's discovery, in 1953, was that it was possible to attach atoms of mercury to particular groups in the haemoglobin molecule. The X-ray diffraction pattern of haemoglobin treated in this way differed from the untreated material. The precise differences proved to pave the way to the final solution of the problem of the three-dimensional structure of haemoglobin.

Myoglobin could not be treated in exactly the same way, but Kendrew found it was possible to prepare five different crystalline compounds of myoglobin containing other heavy atoms. The X-ray diffraction patterns of these were compared with the untreated myoglobin. Solving the problem of the three-dimensional structure of myoglobin from these patterns involved processing tens of millions of numbers, only possible by means of a high speed computer that did not come into use until the late 1950s. Kendrew was the first to make use of such a computer for this type of problem. When this was completed, Kendrew built successively more detailed models of the myoglobin molecule. He had the structure completely resolved by 1960. It was the first protein to have its three-dimensional structure elucidated, and it was the result of outstanding research.

The Herculean task of elucidating the three-dimensional structure of the haemoglobin molecule with its more than 10,000 atoms, took Perutz 23 years, and even then he felt that not every atom had been located! The four polypeptide chains, already known to make up the globin part of the molecule, turned out to be folded in a similar way to those in myoglobin. That knowledge, together with the sequence of the amino acid units along the polypeptide chains, worked out by other scientists in the USA and Germany, combined to give a very good picture of the haemoglobin molecule. Of the four polypeptide chains, two similar α (alpha) chains consist of 141 amino acid units each, and two similar β (beta) chains of 146 amino acid units each. The α and β chains have different sequences of amino acid units, but fold up to form similar three-dimensional structures. Each chain has one haem group with its central atom of iron. The four polypeptide chains lie at the corners of a tetrahedron, but because α and β chains are similar, but not identical chemically, the tetrahedron is not quite regular. Each haem group lies clasped in a fold of the chain, and the whole molecule is practically spherical.

Kendrew worked on myoglobin extracted from the muscle of sperm whale, Perutz on haemoglobin from horse blood. Later work indicated that myoglobin and haemoglobin from other sources have the same three-dimensional structure. As Perutz says, 'It seems as though the apparently haphazard and irregular folding of the chain is a pattern specifically devised for holding a haem group in place and enabling it to carry oxygen'.

In the human there are several normal haemoglobins, haemoglobin A (HbA), is the major one in the adult, with its 2α and 2β chains, but up to 3% of haemoglobin A_2 (HbA$_2$), may be present, with its 2α chains, and 2δ (delta) chains of 146 amino acid units of slightly different composition from the β chains. Haemoglobin F (HbF), is produced in the foetus, and it may represent up to 8% of the total haemoglobin at birth; it has 2α chains, and 2γ (gamma) chains of 146 amino acid units, differing from the β and δ chains. There are a number of abnormal haemoglobins, one will be mentioned later in the chapter.

Human blood forms about 5% of the total body weight. For a body weight of 62.6 kilograms (about 140 lbs), there are about 3 litres of blood. At body temperature, 3 litres of blood without the aid of haemoglobin, would transport no more than $9cm^3$ of oxygen. Haemoglobin increases the oxygen-absorbing capacity 70 times, to enable it to transport $630cm^3$ of oxygen. Haemoglobin, a remarkable compound, so greedy for oxygen, has made the larger animal possible.

As blood passes through the lungs, each of the four atoms of iron in the haemoglobin molecule takes up a molecule of oxygen, and bright red oxyhaemoglobin is formed. During its progress through the tissues oxygen is released, and purplish red deoxyhaemoglobin is formed. The take-up of oxygen by the iron atoms does not involve any change in their divalent (ferrous) state. The capacity of each iron atom to react reversibly with oxygen is a property it acquires through being associated with both haem and globin. Haem alone combines irreversibly with oxygen, the iron atom changing to the trivalent (ferric) state, when it stubbornly holds on to the oxygen it has acquired.

In 1937, Felix Haurowitz had noticed that oxyhaemoglobin formed scarlet needle-shaped crystals whereas deoxyhaemoglobin formed flat hexagonal purple crystals.

He concluded that the two forms represented different molecular structures. Perutz and his co-workers subjected deoxyhaemoglobin to X-ray analysis. Comparison of the results with those for oxyhaemoglobin showed that in the former, the β chains had shifted apart increasing the distance between the iron atoms. Oxyhaemoglobin and deoxyhaemoglobin did indeed have different structures. If samples of blood are exposed to oxygen/nitrogen mixtures with different partial pressures of oxygen, and the percentage saturation of blood with oxygen determined, the results may be plotted on a graph to obtain an oxygen dissociation curve (Figure 7). (The figures in kN/m^2 for the partial pressure of oxygen approximate closely to the percentage of oxygen in the mixture.) The graph shows that as haemoglobin takes up oxygen, its avidity for the gas increases dramatically – it is already 90% saturated when the oxygen concentration is less than 6%. Conversely, as soon as some oxygen is unloaded from the haemoglobin, most of the remainder falls away rapidly.

There is considerable evidence that the progressive increase in affinity for oxygen shown by haemoglobin, corresponds to a change in structure from the form in which the β chains are widely separated (T structure) to the form in which the β chains are closer together (R structure). Unloading of oxygen is related to a change from the R structure back to the T structure.

Why have two oxygen carriers, haemoglobin and

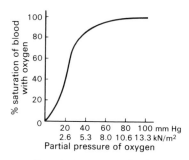

Figure 7 Oxygen dissociation curve for human haemoglobin

myoglobin? Either would become completely saturated with oxygen in the lungs, but whereas oxyhaemoglobin gives up its oxygen readily to tissues that are using up oxygen rapidly, myoglobin, although taking up oxygen even more readily than haemoglobin, will only begin to release it when there is an even greater demand, as in severe muscular exertion. It still has 50% of its oxygen left when haemoglobin, under the same conditions, would have only 2 or 3%. Thus, being present in the muscles, myoglobin acts as an additional oxygen store. Foetal haemoglobin and maternal haemoglobin need to differ in their properties also, for the blood of the foetus has to collect oxygen from the mother's blood across the placenta, and for this to be successful, the foetal haemoglobin needs to have a greater affinity for oxygen than the maternal haemoglobin.

What about the carbon dioxide produced in respiration? It is soluble in water and therefore in plasma, but not soluble enough. It actually combines with water forming a bicarbonate ion and a spare hydrogen ion (proton).

$$CO_2 + H_2O \rightleftharpoons HCO_3^- + H^+$$

Deoxyhaemoglobin behaves as a buffer, it collects up the hydrogen ions, tipping the balance of the reaction towards the formation of bicarbonate ions. Back in the lungs, oxygen molecules push off the hydrogen ions, causing the reaction to go into reverse and forcing carbon dioxide out of the solution to be exhaled.

It was Claude Bernard who showed, in the 19th century, that the poisonous action of carbon monoxide is due to the fact that it takes the place of oxygen in the blood. More recent work shows the affinity of haemoglobin for carbon monoxide is 150 times greater than for oxygen. If you smoke you might like to know that up to 20% of the sites for oxygen take-up in haemoglobin can be blocked by carbon monoxide in tobacco smoke. This not only reduces the capacity of the blood to carry oxygen, but makes it more difficult for the oxygen that is carried to be unloaded in the tissues.

There are more abnormal forms of haemoglobin than there are normal forms. One is associated with the disease of sickle cell anaemia. In 1905, Herrick noted sickle-shaped red blood cells in blood taken from a negro suffering from anaemia. Neel (1949), studied the family histories of individuals suffering from sickle cell anaemia and concluded that it was an hereditary disease. Sufferers were shown to be homozygous for the offending gene: that is, they had inherited a gene for the disease from each parent. Where the gene was inherited from only one parent (the heterozygous condition) there was sickle cell trait, and the blood showed the characteristic sickle shape of the red blood cells only under laboratory conditions of reduced oxygen supply. In the same year, Pauling and his associates showed, by means of electrophoresis, that an abnormal haemoglobin, haemoglobin S (HbS), was present in sufferers from the disease, whereas heterozygous individuals with sickle cell trait, had red blood cells with both haemoglobin S and haemoglobin A. Haemoglobin S is less soluble than haemoglobin A and tends to crystallise as the oxygen concentration falls. This will occur in the tissue capillaries and is the cause of the red blood cells, normally of biconcave disc shape, becoming sickle-shaped. The sickle cells are far less efficient at carrying oxygen and severe anaemia results. Pauling postulated that a mutant or changed gene was responsible for a difference in the structure of the protein of the haemoglobin.

Ingram set out to discover exactly what difference there was between haemoglobin S and haemoglobin A. Using Sanger's method as a basis, he split the globin portion of the haemoglobin into fragments by means of the protein-attacking enzyme, trypsin. It produced 28 peptide chains of about 10 amino acid units each. He subjected these to analysis by electrophoresis and paper chromatography and compared the results. He found that the two haemoglobins differed in one peptide. The sequence of amino acid units in the peptide was then determined and it was found that there was a difference in just one amino acid. In each polypeptide chain, the amino acid, valine, in the haemoglobin S takes the place of the glutamic acid in the normal haemoglobin A. Ingram completed his work in 1956.

Remembering that globin A is made up of 2α and 2β polypeptide chains, and that each α and β chain contains

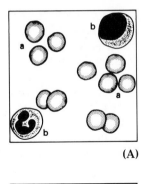

(A)

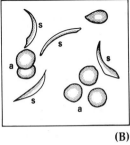

(B)

Figure 8 Human blood, showing (A) normal red cells and (B) sickle cells, abnormal red cells characteristic of sickle cell anaemia. (a = normal red cells, b = white cells, s = sickle cells)

141 and 146 amino acid units respectively, just one amino acid in 287 was found to be responsible for the change from haemoglobin A to haemoglobin S. The slight difference in the haemoglobin caused by such a gene had profound consequences. The gene for haemoglobin S occurs in frequencies as high as 15% in a belt across central Africa, and to some extent in North Africa and round the Mediterranean. One might have expected the sickle cell gene, which in the homozygous state can give rise to anaemia, thrombosis and death, to be eliminated from the population by natural selection, but a very interesting fact came to light. Those with sickle cell trait are able to withstand attacks of the most serious form of malaria (caused by the mosquito-borne parasite *Plasmodium falciparum*) more successfully than

those with normal haemoglobin. Such an advantage leads to the sickle cell gene being retained in populations where malaria is rife.

Chapter 12

Some Advances in Medicine and Surgery

Modern technology, coupled with present knowledge of the blood system, has made possible more accurate diagnosis of vascular problems, and has increased the likelihood of overcoming them by means of up-to-date medical and surgical procedures.

One problem that may arise when there is some degree of insufficiency in the blood supply to the heart, is difficulty in maintaining a smooth and regular heart beat. The heartbeat is initiated by a pacemaker, the sino-auricular node (SAN), lying near the junction of the superior vena cava and the right atrium, and consisting of a plexus of muscle fibres in fibrous tissue. Electrical changes associated with the heartbeat commence in the SAN and radiate over the muscles of the atria and bases of the veins to the junction of the atria and ventricles, stimulating the auriculo-ventricular node (AVN). The wave of electrical disturbance then passes through to the ventricles at the rate of about 500 centimetres a second. Thus all parts of the ventricle contract virtually simultaneously. The progress of the electrical signals can be recorded by means of an electrocardiograph (ECG). If, for some reason, such as an insufficient blood supply, the pathway for the passage of impulses from the SAN is impaired, there may be lack of co-ordination between the contraction of the atria and ventricles. If the impulse from the SAN fails to reach the ventricles, they may respond to signals from the AVN, or to signals arising spontaneously from a pacemaker in the ventricles. The ventricular pacemaker fires too slowly to maintain the normal heartrate, and one result is that the body, as well as the heart itself, it deprived of oxygen and nutrients. If the situation cannot be controlled by suitable drugs, or if the conducting pathways are permanently damaged, an artificial pacemaker may be necessary. Electrodes are introduced into a vein at the base of the neck and coaxed into the heart until they come in contact with the wall of the right ventricle. The electrodes are then connected to a miniature electronic pacemaker implanted under the patient's skin at a suitable point. The pacemaker is a small triumph of electronic engineering.

Once blood transfusion had become a safe procedure, it was possible to contemplate heart surgery; with the development of sophisticated electronic monitoring and other devices, as well as the heart-lung machine, capable of maintaining the patient's circulation and oxygenating the blood, heart surgery became a reality.

In man, changes take place in the inner lining of the arteries that may lead to the formation of soft fatty swellings blocking the free passage of blood – a condition known as atheroma. If the coronary arteries supplying blood to the heart muscle itself are affected, the heart is deprived of essential oxygen and nutrients. The body is remarkably adaptable, however, and if the blockage takes place over a period of time, other vessels may become adapted to carry more blood and bypass the blockage. But, if the roughened surface of a diseased artery causes a blood clot to form, a coronary artery may be suddenly blocked and a 'heart attack' results. In severe cases, one possibility to be considered may be a vein bypass operation. First, some assessment of the extent and severity of the coronary disease will be required. One method of investigation is the coronary angiogram, carried out in the following way: a local anaesthetic is injected into the arm or leg and a wide bore needle is inserted into a major artery. A catheter, or thin flexible tube, is inserted through the needle and coaxed along the artery towards the heart, its progress being monitored on the screen of an X-ray image intensifier. When the catheter is near the heart, a small amount of anticoagulant is injected. Then, when the tip of the catheter is close to each of the coronary arteries in turn, a small amount of radio-opaque dye is injected. The progress of the dye is filmed to enable a permanent record to be made. It will show the outline of the arteries, revealing the presence of any narrowed vessels or blockages.

If a vein bypass operation is decided upon, it will involve removing a length of vein from the patient's leg (the leg can manage quite well without it as there are other veins), and inserting it in front of and beyond the blockage in the coronary artery, perhaps from the origin of the aorta itself, in order to bypass the obstruction. Usually two or three bypasses are inserted at the same time to permit an increased flow of blood to the heart muscle. The patient is put under a general anaesthetic, and the graft is taken from the great saphenous vein that runs from the inside of the ankle to the groin; the branch veins are ligated and a length of vein is removed. Meanwhile, the patient's heart is exposed by cutting along the length of the breastbone, and the blood supply is diverted through a heart-lung machine. A length of healthy coronary artery is exposed and a small slit about one centimetre long is made along its length. The vein for grafting has the end cut diagonally, leaving an elliptical cross section. Then, using a small curved needle and fine thread, it is carefully stitched to the opening in the coronary artery. The vein graft is cut to a suitable length, trimmed by an oblique cut, and stitched to a matching small slit in the aorta. As veins contain valves to prevent backflow of blood, the graft has to be inserted with the valves opening towards the heart. When completed, blood is again allowed to flow along the coronary arteries and the heart will usually begin to beat spontaneously. If it does not, an electric shock will get it going again. The patient is disconnected from the heart-lung machine, and the main incision is closed.

When coronary disease is advanced, it may be impossible by any known medical or surgical means, to get it working efficiently again, and the patient really needs a new one. The big medical problem associated with organ transplants is the rejection of the transplanted organ that the body identifies as foreign tissue. A great deal of research on the immune system of animals and man preceded attempts to transplant organs in the human body.

If a piece of skin is taken from one person and grafted on to another, it is rejected after a few weeks and sloughed off. The tissues of donor and recipient are incompatible. The transplanted skin contains antigens, not present in the recipient, that set his immune response in action. Antibodies are produced and the reaction between antigens and antibodies destroys the cells of the transplanted skin. Before there can be any question of transplanting organs, measures have to be considered for keeping the immune response to a minimum. The most important approach is tissue matching; choosing donor tissue likely to provoke the minimum of immune response, and then treating the patient with drugs designed to suppress the immune response. Unfortunately, these drugs also suppress the response called into play against infecting organisms, and therefore they leave the patient very prone to infection.

The mechanism of the immune response has been the subject of intensive research for at least the last 40 years. The names of a number of well known scientists have been associated with it, notably Sir Peter Medawar, a Nobel Laureate. In 1980, three scientists shared the Nobel Prize for medicine, for their research on the genetical basis of the immunological system. They were George Snell, Jean Dausset, and Baruj Benacerraf.

Snell bred thousands of mice and experimented with transplants between them. The results suggested possible ways in which the mouse recognises its own tissues and rejects foreign tissues. In the 1940s the late Peter Gorer discovered the genetical basis of the rejection of foreign tissue by mice. It was named the H2 system. Snell spent years selectively cross breeding mice to produce inbred strains in which individuals differed only in their H2 type. Mice of the same strain and H2 type would accept grafts from one another, but reject grafts from members of the same strain but different H2 type. While he was establishing his strains, Snell had to test the mice for acceptance or rejection of a skin graft or tumour. Carrying out the test and waiting for the results was tiresome and time consuming.

Bausset discovered the human version of the H2 system, now known as HLA. He found anti-HLA antibodies in people who had, at some time, received foreign blood cells, and this led him to believe that the HLA antigen, causing the antibodies to be produced, was present on blood cells as well as on other cells. This proved to be so. From Dausset's discovery came the development of tissue matching based on a blood test, making it fairly simple to find out if a proposed organ transplant stands a chance of being accepted. Dausset found that a gene complex is concerned in the HLA system, and it is now known that the number of different HLA types is very large indeed. Landsteiner believed that blood would be found to be as individual as a fingerprint, and he may well prove to be right.

Following the discovery that the HLA genes control the production of antigens carried on the surface of cells, Benacerraf hoped to find out how the body recognised them and brought about the rejection of tissue. He and his co-workers discovered that the genes in command of the immune system (Ir genes), lie within the HLA complex. An Ir gene will instruct a certain type of white blood cell (T cell), to react with the foreign antigen. An unexpected development of Benacerraf's work was the detection of a relationship between the HLA system and some human diseases, for example, rheumatoid arthritis and multiple sclerosis. This opened up a very promising line of research.

Some understanding of the tissue rejection mechanism in man, the development of methods of tissue matching from blood samples, and the availability of immunosuppressive drugs, provided the necessary background for attempts at organ transplants, first carried out on man with kidneys, with increasing degrees of success. For patients who had previously been obliged to spend many hours a week attached to a dialysis machine to remove waste from the blood, it seemed like a miracle.

One morning, in December 1967, the world awoke to find that in Cape Town, a patient, Louis Washkansky, had been supplied with a new heart. The surgeon responsible for this achievement was Christiaan Barnard.

Christiaan Barnard was born in 1922, and studied medicine at the University of Cape Town. For a while (1948–51), he was in private practice before appointments, successively, as Senior Resident Medical Officer at the City Hospital in Cape Town (1951–53); Registrar at the Groote Schurr Hospital; and Registrar of the Surgery Department at the University of Cape Town. The Charles Adams Memorial Scholarship and a bursary took him to the USA for further study. There he was awarded a public health grant for research in cardiac surgery, and in 1958, he gained further degrees from the University of Minnesota. He returned to Cape Town as a specialist cardio-thoracic surgeon, and by 1961 he was Head of Cardio-Thoracic Surgery at the Cape Town University Teaching Hospitals, and an Associate Professor of the University in the following year. Barnard has been awarded numerous honorary doctorates, foreign orders and awards. He is a member of a number of learned societies, author of technical and popular books and an active contributor to scientific journals.

The heart transplant was a surgical triumph for which Christiaan Barnard is justly famous. Since that time the operation has been performed at other centres in Britain; at the Papworth Hospital in Cambridge, and at the Harefield Hospital in Middlesex. Not surprisingly, it has raised many problems, ethical as well as medical.

The early heart transplants required two teams of surgeons working in adjoining operating theatres. In one, surgeons prepared the patient to receive the organ transplant, while in the other, the surgical team removed the heart from the body of the donor whose heart and lungs had been kept functioning after death, by means of a respirator. Later it was found possible to keep a donor heart in good condition for several hours after removal, to enable it to be transported to the hospital where the transplant was to take place. First, after removal, the donor heart is washed in dilute salt solution containing heparin, an anti-clotting agent, then placed in a sterile bag containing dilute salt solution and packed round with ice. Meanwhile, the patient is prepared to receive the donor organ. After opening the chest cavity and freeing the heart from the protective membrane, the pericardium, the patient is connected to a heart-lung machine. The vena cavae, the vessels returning blood from the systemic circulation to the right atrium, are not severed but detached together by cutting out a small piece of atrium wall to which they are connected. The pulmonary veins, vessels returning blood from the lungs to the left atrium are detached together in a similar way. Removal of the old heart in this way makes attachment of the donor heart a simpler process, for stitching in the cup-shaped pieces of atrium with their attached blood vessels is easier and speedier than suturing individual blood vessels. When circulation to the new heart is restored and the heart warmed, heartbeat may start of its own accord, if not, a single electric shock will start it. The patient is taken off the heart-lung machine and the new heart takes over the circulation. With the confidence of the great, Christiaan Barnard tells us 'The operation is a very simple one'.

Barnard is the first to acknowledge his debt to a number of scientists who worked on organ transplants in animals, from Alexis Carrel, a French-American surgeon who developed the technique of suturing blood vessels, to the Russian surgeon, Demikhov, who transplanted the hearts of dogs, with short-term success.

The major medical problem associated with heart transplants is rejection of the donor heart. By careful tissue matching of donor and recipient, the possibility of rejection may be minimised. Drugs suppress the reduced immune reaction, but care must be taken to protect the patient from infection, for these drugs also impair the patient's ability to combat invading organisms. Research is in progress to develop a more specific immunosuppressive material which will not interfere with the patient's response to infecting organisms.

Since 1945, blood transfusion has become of increasing importance owing to the development of many new medical and surgical procedures. More recently, since about 1965, it has been possible not merely to separate whole blood into cells and plasma, but to separate plasma itself into different dissolved protein fractions. Whole blood is used where blood volume and oxygen-carrying capacity need to be replaced, as for example, following blood loss during surgery, or severe haemorrhage. It is also used to supplement the circulation during cardiac surgery. For replacement of blood volume, the albumin fraction from plasma may be used, but where the oxygen-carrying capacity is depleted, a concentrate of red blood cells may be employed.

The Blood Products Laboratory, at Elstree, currently processes all the blood plasma supplied by the regional transfusion centres in England and Wales, and there is a Protein Fractionation Centre in Edinburgh. The British Pharmacopoeia, Volume 2 (1980), lists 16 blood products, most of which are not available commercially, but which are obtainable for medical use and research. The products include whole blood, mixed with an anticoagulant and tested for freedom from syphilitic and hepatitis B infections; a concentrate of red blood cells, and plasma. Various plasma fractions are prepared, including albumin; and those fractions which are rich in clotting factors; are of use in the treatment of haemophilia, a severe and often fatal disease in which, owing to the failure of the blood to clot, a minor injury may prove disastrous. Preparations are also produced from plasma to treat a number of dangerous diseases such as tetanus, rabies and smallpox. (The World Health Organisation has now declared the world free of smallpox, but the relevant preparation will probably continue to be available at key centres in the world for some time.) Each of these preparations contains human globulins with antibodies specific to the disease, prepared from the pooled plasma of a large number of donors, 1000 in some cases, who have been immunised against the disease. Additionally, a preparation of human globulins is available containing antibodies of normal adults – this is used to boost general disease resistance. Other preparations include dried thrombin and fibrinogen, separate blood clotting factors, and one of the incomplete antibodies against the Rhesus antigen of human red blood cells.

It may come as a surprise that there is such a product as artificial blood. Not 'whole blood' with its complex cells, coagulating factors, antibodies and so on, but an artificial oxygen-carrying fluid, a substitute haemoglobin-in-solution, not blood-red in colour, but white. Artificial blood is a perfluorochemical compound in the form of an emulsion. Perfluorochemicals are like fluorocarbons with all the hydrogen atoms replaced by fluorine. Gases such as oxygen and carbon dioxide dissolve in them. In the form of an emulsion, they appear to be harmless when administered intravenously, and are said to have saved lives. It is not easy to believe that artificial blood has a great future, but time will tell.

Chapter 13

Blood Biochemistry – a Modern Research Tool

Geographical distribution of races

Once Landsteiner had announced his discovery of the ABO blood groups, it was not long before it was found that the groups occur in different proportions in different populations. The ABO groups are insufficient to distinguish separate races, but when considered in conjunction with other groups, particularly the M, N and Rhesus groups, blood typing assumes greater significance.

This finding fired the imagination of William Boyd, an American biochemist. He was born in Missouri in 1903, graduated from Harvard University and gained his doctorate at Boston. He joined the staff of the Boston University School of Medicine and remained there until his retirement. William Boyd and his wife travelled extensively during the 1930s for the purpose of blood typing populations. In 1956, from the data they collected, together with the results of surveys undertaken by others, Boyd was able to divide man into five major divisions, each capable of being subdivided, giving a total of 13 sub-groups. The five major divisions are, European (Caucasoids), African (Negroids), American Indian, Asiatic (Mongoloids), and Pacific (Australoids). The divisions are in broad agreement with those made on the basis of external physical characters, such as skin colour, type and colour of hair, eye colour, shape of head, and so on. In his book *Genetics and the Races of Man*, William Boyd points out that the genetic classification of races is more objective and better founded scientifically than classification based on external characters. He makes a point against racial prejudice in his comment, '. . . since we have absolutely no reason to think that the possession or lack of any of the genes we have considered here (i.e. those concerning blood groups) confers on the possessor any advantage as a potential contributor to the advance of cultures and civilisations, there is no reason that any prejudice should exist.' One of Boyd's interesting findings was the existence of an early European race, characterised by a high frequency of the Rhesus negative blood group. It was displaced by the modern Caucasoids, but is still found in the western Pyrenees. We know this group as the Basques. Boyd's main divisions distinguish the populations of continents, a finding that agrees with the theory that geographical isolation leads to differentiation of a species into races.

Tracing the routes of migration taken by ancient peoples, or even those that have taken place in more modern times, is sometimes made possible by a study of blood group frequencies. Inhabitants of central Asia have the highest incidence of blood group B, which decreases rapidly both to the west and the east. Its occurrence in Western Europe is probably due to an invasion by Huns in the 5th century AD, or the Mongolians in the 13th century AD, or both.

Chemical paleogenetics. A new method of constructing evolutionary history

Haemoglobin and myoglobin are believed to have had a common molecular ancestor about 650 million years ago. This would date back to the Precambrian period, millions of years before the earliest vertebrates appeared. The basis for this belief lies in the work of Emile Zuckerkandl and Linus Pauling. Zuckerkandl reasoned that if in human haemoglobins the polypeptide chains have the same function, the same configuration, and a considerable proportion of identical amino acid units occurring at corresponding molecular sites, it seems reasonable to suppose they have a common molecular ancestor. When the α chain of adult human haemoglobin with its 141 amino acid units is compared with the β chain with its 146 amino acid units, it is found that they have 64 sites where the amino acids are the same. Their many differences, however, suggest that they diverged from a common ancestor long ago. The β, γ and δ polypeptide chains all have 146 amino acid units, but there are only 39 differences between β and γ chains and a mere 10 differences between β and δ.

It is possible to get some idea of how long ago these different forms diverged from a common molecular ancestor. Four animals were selected, known, from other evidence, to have had a common ancestor with man about 80 million years ago. The α polypeptide chains of their haemoglobins, and the β chains, where appropriate, were compared with the corresponding chains in man, and the number of sites where the amino acid units differed was noted. Calculation showed the mean number of differences to be 22, or an average of 11 changes in each chain. If then, the common ancestor of man and these animals lived 80 million years ago, the average time needed for a successful amino acid change to be established would be 80/11 or about 7 million years.

Returning to the problem of the human haemoglobins armed with this piece of information, it is possible to estimate how long ago it was that the four polypeptide chains, occurring in human haemoglobins, had a common molecular ancestor. β and δ polypeptide chains are most alike with 10 differences, or 5 in each chain. If one change takes 7 million years, then they must have diverged about 35 million years ago. The β and γ chains have 39 differences or approximately 20 in each chain, while α and β have 76 differences or 38 per chain. But, as Zuckerkandl points out, the greater the number of differences between two chains, the greater are the chances that a change may have occurred at a particular site more than once. Linus Pauling made allowance for this possibility in further calculations. They point to the divergence of β and γ chains about 150 million years ago, and the divergence of α and β chains 380 million years ago.

This method of analysis, chemical paleogenetics, has been used to investigate the degree of relationship between, for example, a number of mammals. It provides a new method of constructing evolutionary history.

Blood and crime

Modern knowledge of the physical and chemical character-
istics of blood is of inestimable value in the detection of
crime. Not only is it possible to distinguish human blood
from animal blood, but sophisticated methods of analysis
can reveal secrets of the ABO, Rhesus and other blood
groups from the smallest blood spot or smear. It may even
be possible to determine a criminal's blood group without
any blood at all, for in addition to being found on red blood
cells, the antigens A, B and H are present in other tissues
and, in 50% of Europeans, in body fluids such as saliva and
tears. The H antigen is found in all human red blood cells,
and is a kind of parent substance from which antigens A
and B are produced. The quantity varies according to the
blood group, but most is found in blood group O, where,
of course, antigens A and B are absent. Examination of the
gum on a used envelope might reveal, for example, that the
sender was of blood group AB, if antigens A, B and H were
detected. Individuals bearing antigens in the body fluids
are called secretors. In fact they have two forms of antigen,
an alcohol soluble form in the cells and a water soluble form
in the secretions, while non-secretors lack the water soluble
form. The presence or absence of A, B and H antigens in
secretions is controlled by a pair of alleles, Se and se, their
inheritance being independent of the ABO system.

Cases of disputed paternity

Information about the blood group of a mother, her child
and that of the putative father, together with a knowledge
of the method of inheritance of blood groups, may be used
in solving cases of disputed paternity. Clearly, if the child
carries a gene not present in the mother then it must have
been inherited from the father. If the putative father does
not have the gene then he cannot be the real father. Consider a case in which Mr. T. is said to be the father of baby
John. The mother is blood group O, the baby blood group
A, and Mr. T. of blood group B. Mr. T. cannot be the father
of John, for the gene for A must have come from the father.
In another case, baby Ann of blood group O was born to a
mother also of blood group O. Mr. X. said to be the father

is of blood group AB. He cannot be the father for he must donate either a gene for A or for B to his offspring. In a third case, baby Jane is of blood group B, her mother of blood group A. The baby is believed to have been fathered by Mr. G. who is of blood group B. He could be Jane's father, but any other man of blood group B could equally well have been the father, and so could any man of blood group AB. A blood group may be used to establish innocence, but alone it is insufficient to establish guilt. It is fortunate if the ABO group alone is sufficient to establish innocence, otherwise additional groups such as the Rhesus and M and N, may have to be considered.

Glossary

Active immunity   Antibodies produced in the blood as the result of the introduction of antigens in the form of dead or weakened disease organisms constituting the vaccine.

Agglutination   The sticking together of red blood cells when mixed with incompatible blood, or the sticking together of bacteria brought about by antibodies.

Alleles   Contrasting forms of a gene.

Angiogram   X-ray film of blood vessels injected with radio-opaque substance to demonstrate any narrowing of the vessels.

Antibody   Substance produced in the blood to combine with invading antigen.

Antigen   Substance foreign to the body, often protein in nature, capable of initiating antibody formation.

Antitoxin   A type of antibody produced in the blood neutralising poisonous waste (toxin) produced by some microorganisms.

Aorta   The main artery.

Artery   Thick-walled blood vessel carrying oxygenated blood from the heart. (See pulmonary artery)

Atrium   One of the two smaller chambers of the heart.

Bicuspid valve   Valve between the atrium and the ventricle on the left side of the heart.

Blood cells/corpuscles   The non-liquid part of the blood.

Blood letting   Practice of opening a vein or scratching the skin to allow blood to flow in belief it was of benefit to patient.

Capillary   The smallest blood vessel found between artery and vein.

Chemotherapy   Treatment of disease by chemical methods.

Chromosome   Microscopic thread (of DNA and protein) consisting of units, the genes, appearing in the nucleus during cell division.

Comparative anatomy   Study of the similarities and differences in the anatomy of different animals.

Coronary vessels   Vessels taking blood to and from the heart muscle.

Diastole   Phase of the heart beat when the heart muscle is relaxed and the heart is filling with blood.

Dominant gene   The one with the most influence in a pair of alleles.

Ductus arteriosus   Blood vessel in foetus joining pulmonary artery to aorta, allowing blood to by-pass lungs.

Electrocardiograph (ECG)   Instrument for recording variations in electrical potential occurring in the heart. Used for diagnosis of possible heart disorders.

Electrocardiogram (ECG)   Tracing produced on the electrocardiograph.

Embryology   Study of the development of embryos.

Endoderm   Layer of cells in animal embryo developing into the gut and associated glands.

Entomology   Study of insects.

Foramen ovale   Opening between atria in foetal heart allowing portion of oxygenated blood from the placenta returning to the right atrium to go straight to the left atrium and thence to the left ventricle and aorta while lungs are non-functional.

Gene   Unit of a chromosome responsible for a particular character in an organism.

Genotype   The genetic make-up of an organism.

Haemoglobin   A red pigment in the red blood cells having a high affinity for oxygen.

Heterozygous   Having two contrasting genes for the same character.

Homeostasis   Maintenance of a steady state in the internal environment of the body.

Homozygous   Having two similar genes for the same character.

Immunology   Study of the ability of an organism to resist disease.

Immunity   Protection from a disease conferred by the presence in the body of specific antibodies ready to react with invading antigens associated with the disease.

Interventricular septum   Muscular wall separating the ventricles of the heart.

Mesoderm   Layer of cells in animal embryo developing into blood, muscles, connective tissue etc.

Myoglobin   A substance occuring in muscle fibres, closely-related to haemoglobin, and having an even greater affinity for oxygen.

Ophthalmology   Study of the eye and its diseases.

Passive immunity   Immunity achieved by injecting into the body antibodies which have been produced in another animal.

Pericardium   Membranous sac enclosing the heart.

Plasma   Liquid part of the blood.

Platelet   Minute body in the blood concerned in blood clotting.

Pulmonary artery   Artery carrying *deoxygenated* blood from the right ventricle of the heart to the lungs.

Pulmonary vein   Vein carrying *oxygenated* blood from the lungs to the left atrium of the heart.

Recessive gene   The one with the least influence in a pair of alleles.

Rhesus factor   An antigen present in the red blood cells of 85% of the population in Britain (Rhesus positive), and absent in the remainder (Rhesus negative). The Rhesus negative genotype is distributed mainly in north-west Europe.

Semi-lunar valve   Crescent-shaped valve at the base

of the aorta and the base of the pulmonary artery preventing backflow of blood into the heart.

Serum   Blood plasma without the clotting agents.

Sino-auricular node (SAN)   The heart's pacemaker.

Systole   Phase of the heart beat when the heart muscle is contracted and blood is being pumped into the arteries.

Toxin   Poisonous substance produced by microorganisms stimulating the production of a neutralising substance (antitoxin) in the body.

Trepanning/Trephining   Operation in which a portion of the skull bone is removed.

Tricuspid valve   Valve between the atrium and ventricle on the right side of the heart.

Vaccine   Preparation of dead or weakened microorganisms for inoculation, capable of stimulating the production of antibodies resulting in immunity to the disease.

Vascular system   Blood system in animals.

Vein   Blood vessel with valves at intervals returning deoxygenated blood to the heart. (See pulmonary vein)

Vena cava   The vena cavae are the main veins in the body.

Venesection   Blood letting.

Ventricle   One of the two larger chambers of the heart.

Select Bibliography

Anderson, I. *Heart Attack* (Macmillan, 1980)

Barnard, C. *Heart Attack* (Allen, 1973)

Boyd, W. C. *Genetics and Races of Man* (Boston, Little, Brown & Co, 1950)

Calder, R. *Leonardo* (Heinemann, 1970)

Casson, L. *Ancient Egypt* (Time-Life International, 1969)

Cheetham, N. *New Spain: The Birth of Modern Mexico* (Gollancz, 1974)

Clarke, C. A. *The Prevention of Rhesus Babies, Scientific American* 219 (5) p. 46 1968

Cockayne, O. *Leechdoms, Wortcunning and Starcraft of Early England* 3 vols. (Rolls Series, London 1864–6) (Delightful books to dip into)

Cole, S. *Races of Man* (British Museum, natural history, 1965)

Crispens, C. G. *Essentials of Medical Genetics* (Harper and Row, 1971)

Franklin, K. J. *Translation of William Harvey's Movement of the Heart and Blood in Animals* (Oxford, 1957)

Inglis, B. *A History of Medicine* (Weidenfeld and Nicholson, 1965)

Keele, K. *Leonardo da Vinci and the Art of Science* (Priory Press, 1977)

Keele, K. *William Harvey* (Nelson, 1965)

Kendrew, J. *The Three-Dimensional Structure of a Protein Molecule (i.e. myoglobin), Scientific American* 205 (6) 1961

Keynes, G. *The Life of William Harvey* (Oxford, 1966)

Kramer, S. N. *Cradle of Civilisation* (Time-Life International, 1969)

Leonard, J. N. *Ancient America* (Time-Life International, 1970)

Mackean, D. G. *Introduction to Biology* (Murray, 1973) (Good background reading on the blood, circulation and heart, and on genetics.)

Neil, E. *William Harvey and the Circulation of the Blood* (Priory Press, 1975)

Perutz, M. F. *The Haemoglobin Molecule, Scientific American* 211 (5) p. 64 1964

Perutz, M. F. *Haemoglobin Structure and Respiratory Transport, Scientific American* 239 (6) p. 92 1978

Reid, R. *Microbes and Men* (B.B.C, 1974)

Roberts, M. B. V. *Biology. A Functional Approach* (Nelson, 1971) (Good background reading – more advanced than Mackean.)

Rose, M. *Artificial Blood – An Emergency Airlift?, New Scientist* 88 (1229) p. 562 1980

Rubin, S. *Medieval English Medicine* (David and Charles, 1974)

Stewart, D. *Early Islam* (Time-Life International, 1969)

Vallentin, A. *Leonardo da Vinci: The Tragic Pursuit of Perfection* (Allen, 1952)

Venzmer, G. *5000 Years of Medicine* (Macdonald, 1972)

Von Hagen, W. *The Ancient Sun Kingdoms of the Americas* (Thames and Hudson, 1962, Panther Edition, 1967)

Zuckerkandl, E. *The Evolution of Haemoglobin, Scientific American* 212 (5) p. 110 1965

Index